Practical Problems and Approaches in Genetic Counseling

This innovative text aims to help the genetic counselor in training and in practice prepare for the challenges arising in everyday patient scenarios, spanning genomic medicine, communication challenges, ethical issues, and emerging topics in a fast-moving field.

- Advises the practitioner on how to pre-empt and tackle problem topics in genetic counseling practice
- Tackles new and emerging challenges arising in everyday clinical scenarios
- Presents precise and targeted advice in an approachable style

Priyanka R. Ahimaz, MS, CGC, is an Associate Professor of Genetic Counseling in Pediatrics, Columbia University, New York, NY. She has more than 15 years of experience in clinical care, research, and education. She has a strong interest in research with direct clinical relevance to patient-centered care and is passionate about expanding access to genetic counseling. She is particularly focused on efforts to empower healthcare providers in primary and specialty medicine to integrate genetic counseling into their practice. With a keen interest in identifying and responding to emerging trends in genetic counseling, she actively works to anticipate changes in the field and adapt clinical and educational strategies to stay ahead. She has held leadership positions overseeing clinical genetic counseling practices, supervising students and their research, and managing educational programs, as well as serving in leadership roles within national professional organizations, including the National Society of Genetic Counselors (NSGC) and the American Board of Genetic Counseling (ABGC).

Practical Problems and Approaches in Genetic Counseling

Challenges in the Era of Genomic Medicine

Edited by
Priyanka R. Ahimaz, MS, CGC

Associate Professor of Genetic Counseling in Pediatrics
Columbia University
New York, New York

CRC Press
Taylor & Francis Group
Boca Raton London New York

CRC Press is an imprint of the
Taylor & Francis Group, an **informa** business

Designed cover image: Shutterstock

First edition published 2026
by CRC Press
2385 NW Executive Center Drive, Suite 320, Boca Raton, FL 33431

and by CRC Press
4 Park Square, Milton Park, Abingdon, Oxon, OX14 4RN

CRC Press is an imprint of Taylor & Francis Group, LLC

© 2026 selection and editorial matter, Priyanka Ahimaz; individual chapters, the contributors

ISBN: 978-1-032-50302-8 (hbk)
ISBN: 978-1-032-49566-8 (pbk)
ISBN: 978-1-003-39784-7 (ebk)

DOI: 10.1201/9781003397847

Typeset in Caslon
by Apex CoVantage, LLC

Contents

PREFACE   vii

CONTRIBUTORS   ix

CHAPTER 1   VARIANTS OF UNCERTAIN SIGNIFICANCE: VARIANT
CURATION AND INTERPRETATION   1

ANYA REVAH-POLITI

CHAPTER 2   THE ROLE OF RACE, ETHNICITY, AND ANCESTRY
IN GENOMIC TESTING   8

AISHWARYA ARJUNAN, KATELYNN G. SAGASER, AND
SALLY A. RODRIGUEZ

CHAPTER 3   RESEARCH GENETIC TESTING   15

NATALIE C. LIPPA

CHAPTER 4   CHALLENGING THE NORM OF NONDIRECTIVE COUNSELING   21

ERICA SPIEGEL

CHAPTER 5   LOSS AND GRIEF IN THE ERA OF GENOMIC MEDICINE   28

AMANDA L. BERGNER

CHAPTER 6   COUNTERTRANSFERENCE   37

MICHELLE E. FLORIDO

CHAPTER 7   CHALLENGES TO STUDENT TRAINING IN THE GENOMIC ERA   44

ELANA LEVINSON

CHAPTER 8   COMMUNICATION AND DOCUMENTATION IN THE
ELECTRONIC HEALTH RECORD   51

SARA M. BERGER

CHAPTER 9 OBTAINING CONSENT WITH INTERPRETERS 57
NINA HARKAVY

CHAPTER 10 GENETIC TESTING FOR MINORS 63
MARGARET B. MENZEL

CHAPTER 11 OBTAINING CONSENT IN ACUTE SETTINGS 68
MICHELE DISCO

CHAPTER 12 ETHICAL ISSUES WITH OBTAINING CONSENT FOR
PREDICTIVE GENETIC TESTING 74
JILL S. GOLDMAN

CHAPTER 13 EMERGING SPECIALTIES IN GENETIC COUNSELING:
A PATH TOWARDS THE FUTURE OF GENETIC COUNSELING 80
NATALIE VENA

CHAPTER 14 EXPANDED CARRIER SCREENING AND NEWBORN
SCREENING 87
JOSIE PERVOLA, CHARLOTTE CLOSE, AND
ALEXANDRA DEMERS

CHAPTER 15 NAVIGATING NEW FRONTIERS: WHAT GENETIC
COUNSELORS NEED TO KNOW ABOUT GENETIC
THERAPIES AND CLINICAL TRIALS 94
LOUISE BIER AND HETANSHI NAIK

CHAPTER 16 ARTIFICIAL INTELLIGENCE AND THE FUTURE OF
GENOMIC MEDICINE 101
SHIVANI B. NAZARETH

INDEX 109

Preface

Over the course of my career in genetic counseling, one constant has remained: change. As genetic counselors, we are often at the intersection of rapidly changing science and deeply personal patient experiences – which is something I love and cherish about our profession. The field has evolved in many ways that were once unimaginable, driven by advancements in genomic sequencing technologies, the accessibility of genomic testing, and the expanding scope of precision medicine. These shifts bring incredible opportunities for genetic counselors as well as unprecedented challenges to offering humanistic patient care that require innovative solutions. This guidebook – *Practical Problems and Approaches in Genetic Counseling: Challenges in the Era of Genomic Medicine* – was born from this ever-present evolution and aims to provide practical insights to navigate genetic counseling challenges seen in the genomic era. The content in this guidebook emerged from years of clinical practice observations, engaging case discussions with peers, and a desire to share collective wisdom and practical knowledge from fieldwork.

In the first section, authors explore the limitations and ambiguities inherent in genomic analysis, including the interpretation of variants of uncertain significance, incidental findings, integral differences between research and clinical genomic testing, and the relevance of race, ancestry, and ethnicity in the genomic era. We address how genetic counselors can manage these uncertainties and guide patients through the complexities of genomic data.

The second section delves into modern communication challenges genetic counselors face in their jobs as clinicians and educators. Effective communication in this context goes beyond the technical; it requires cultural competence, emotional intelligence, and the ability to adapt to the diverse needs of patients, students, and colleagues. Through real-world case studies and evidence-based strategies, we aim to provide tools for enhancing communication skills and fostering an inclusive, supportive environment for both patients and trainees.

Ethical considerations are at the heart of genetic counseling, particularly in the context of informed consent. As such, the third section addresses the unique dilemmas associated with obtaining truly informed consent for genomic testing for diverse patient populations. It provides frameworks for navigating these ethical challenges, emphasizing best practices for fostering informed decision-making and respecting patient autonomy. These chapters encourage reflection on how we can make our practices more inclusive, responsive, and equitable – hallmarks of a field that continues to evolve alongside the science.

The final section explores emerging trends, including the integration of artificial intelligence in genomic medicine, the role of genetic counselors in clinical trials and therapeutics, the evolving landscape of genetic counseling in different specialized fields, and the emergence of genomic medicine in public health. As the field continues to expand, genetic counselors must remain adaptable, continuously updating their knowledge and skill sets to remain effective in guiding patients and healthcare providers through the genomic revolution. These forward-looking chapters aim to inspire curiosity, agility, and a proactive mindset – traits that will be essential as we collectively shape the future of our profession.

I am deeply grateful to the experts and visionaries who contributed their knowledge and insights to this project. Their contributions are invaluable in ensuring that this book reflects the latest thinking in the field, and their expertise is evident in every chapter. Their willingness to share their experiences and lessons learned makes this book not just a collection of information, but a resource for anyone practicing genetic counseling. This guidebook is intended for both seasoned genetic counselors and those entering the field, offering a comprehensive overview of current challenges and forward-looking solutions. By addressing these critical issues, we aim to empower genetic counselors to navigate the evolving complexities of the current era with confidence and insight. We hope this book serves as a valuable resource in your practice and encourages thoughtful discussion about the future of genetic counseling in the genomic age.

Priyanka R. Ahimaz
New York, New York

Contributors

Aishwarya Arjunan
GRAIL, Inc.
Menlo Park, CA

Sara M. Berger
Department of Pediatrics
Irving Medical Center
Columbia University
New York, NY

Amanda L. Bergner
Department of Genetics & Development
Department of Neurology
Vagelos College of Physicians & Surgeons
Columbia University
New York, NY

Louise Bier
Genetics & Genomic Sciences
Icahn School of Medicine at Mount Sinai
New York, NY

Charlotte Close
Genetic Counseling in Pediatrics
Columbia University
New York, NY

Alexandra Demers
Genetic Counseling in Obstetrics &
   Gynecology
Columbia University
New York, NY

Michele Disco
Division of Clinical Genetics
Columbia University
New York, NY

Michelle E. Florido
Department of Genetics & Development
Columbia University
New York, NY

Jill S. Goldman
Department of Neurology
Irving Medical Center
Columbia University
New York, NY

Nina Harkavy
Vagelos College of Physicians & Surgeons
Columbia University
New York, NY

Elana Levinson
Division of Digestive & Liver Diseases
Irving Medical Center
Columbia University
New York, NY

Natalie C. Lippa
Genetic Counseling in Medicine
Department of Cardiology
Columbia University
New York, NY

Margaret B. Menzel
George Washington University School
   of Medicine & Health Sciences
Washington, DC

Hetanshi Naik
Department of Genetics
Stanford University School of Medicine
Palo Alto, CA

Shivani B. Nazareth
Digital Health Strategy
Myriad Genetics
New York, NY

Josie Pervola
Department of Obstetrics & Gynecology
Columbia University
New York, NY

Anya Revah-Politi
Genetic Counseling in Neurology
Columbia University
New York, NY

Sally A. Rodriguez
Laboratory Genetic Services
Sequence46, LLC
Los Angeles, CA

Katelynn G. Sagaser
Exact Sciences Corporation
Madison, WI

Erica Spiegel
Genetic Counseling in Obstetrics &
   Gynecology
Columbia University
New York, NY

Natalie Vena
Department of Medicine
Columbia University
New York, NY

VARIANTS OF UNCERTAIN SIGNIFICANCE

Variant Curation and Interpretation

ANYA REVAH-POLITI

Introduction

Recent advancements in high-throughput next-generation sequencing have led to a surge in complex genetic testing, presenting new challenges in variant interpretation. To address this, the American College of Medical Genetics (ACMG), the Association for Molecular Pathology (AMP), and the College of American Pathologists (CAP) released standards and guidelines in 2015 known as the "ACMG/AMP criteria." These guidelines, still used by clinical laboratories today, replaced the terms "mutation" and "polymorphism" with "variant" and suggested modifiers: pathogenic, likely pathogenic, uncertain significance, likely benign, or benign.

These guidelines provide two sets of criteria: one for the classification of pathogenic or likely pathogenic variants and one for the classification of benign or likely benign variants. If a variant does not meet criteria using either of these sets or the evidence is conflicting, it is classified as a variant of uncertain significance (VUS). The guidelines describe pieces of evidence including inheritance pattern, variant type, types of variants that are disease-causing and their location within the gene, presence of the variant in control databases and affected individuals, functional studies, genic intolerance, and *in silico* predictors, among others. For more details on the strength and combination of these evidence types, refer to Richards et al. (2015).

Despite these guidelines, inconsistencies in variant classification persist among laboratories. To address this, the Clinical Genome Resource (ClinGen) established the Sequence Variant Interpretation Working Group (SVI WG), which publishes the "ClinGen Recommendations for Using ACMG/AMP Criteria" on the ClinGen website. Their aim is to reduce subjectivity by developing quantitative approaches to specific pieces of evidence, which allow for their upgrading or downgrading. The increased stringency of the ClinGen Recommendations results in a larger number of variants being classified as VUSs.

DOI: 10.1201/9781003397847-1

Challenges and Strategies

Discrepancies between Laboratory Classifications

Discrepancies in how different laboratories classify a variant may occur due to incorrect/outdated application of the classification guidelines, curator subjectivity, or the use of internal or unpublished data. Curating and classifying variants requires significant infrastructure, and while some processes can be automated, a manual review of the variant is still required. Because there are no standards across laboratories about what should be reported, some laboratories may report more VUSs than others. When choosing a laboratory to send testing to, it is essential to read the fine print about what they will and will not report.

There is also no consensus about who is responsible for requesting the reinterpretation of a variant (the laboratory, the clinical team, or the client). If a variant needs reassessment, contacting the laboratory's director or genetic counselor is recommended to discuss reinterpretation. If a significant amount of time has passed since the initial test, it may be more effective to consider newer technologies such as exome or genome sequencing (ES/GS) instead of reinterpreting a single variant.

Researching a Variant

Following is a list of strategies to consider when researching a variant.

a. Reference Genome Build and Gene Transcripts

- When researching a variant, make sure you identify the reference genome build and the gene transcript used to describe the variant. This information can be found in the laboratory report.
- The human genome reference build corresponds to the version of the complete nucleotide sequences used for comparing samples and identifying genomic variants. GRCh37/hg19 and GRCh38/hg38 are two commonly used versions. The Broad Institute's Lift Over Tool can convert variants between these versions (link in Bibliography).
- The gene transcript number is crucial for accurate variant identification and starts with ENST (if using the Ensembl genome browser) or NM_ (if using the NCBI Reference Sequence, or Refseq). Different publications may use different transcripts, so it is essential to confirm the transcript to ensure accurate variant identification in the literature. Tools such as Variant Effect Predictor, Varsome, and Franklin (links in Bibliography) provide details on a variant across various transcripts. If possible, double-check the variant's genomic coordinate to prevent errors due to transcript discrepancies.

b. Useful Databases

- ClinGen is an NIH-funded central resource on the clinical relevance of genes and variants. It has several Curation Working Groups on topics such as gene–disease validity, clinical actionability, and variant pathogenicity. ClinGen's findings are regularly updated by expert panels, making it a highly reliable resource for variant interpretation.
- Public databases like ClinVar and subscription-based resources like the Human Gene Mutation Database (HGMD) help determine if a variant has been reported in affected individuals and its classification. However, entries in these databases may not be peer-reviewed, and critical evaluation of the evidence listed is essential.
- Public control population databases such as the Genome Aggregation Database (gnomAD) and the Trans-Omics for Precision Medicine (TOPMed) Program are crucial for determining whether the variant of interest has been seen in the "healthy" control population. Note that disease-causing variants may be present in these databases because of variable expressivity, reduced penetrance, late age of disease onset, somatic mosaicism, and because the condition is recessive. It is also more likely that variants in individuals from non-European ancestry groups will be absent in control databases, which reflects the underrepresentation of these populations in these databases, an issue continuously being addressed.

c. Family Studies

- Determining whether a variant is inherited or *de novo* can be useful in evaluating VUSs. Testing biological parents (if available) is often the most informative place to start.
- A *de novo* variant without a family history of the same phenotype may be upgraded to likely pathogenic. Caveats include whether maternity and paternity are confirmed or assumed. In a more recent ClinGen Recommendation, phenotypic specificity, genetic heterogeneity of the phenotype, confirmation of parental relationships, and number of *de novo* observations in the literature can be used to downgrade or upgrade the evidence.
- An inherited or familial variant is less likely to be upgraded to likely pathogenic even if it segregates with disease within a family. Since there is a 50% prior probability that the variant is inherited from either parent, its presence in an affected parent does not increase the likelihood that it is disease-causing, especially in conditions with high genetic heterogeneity. Segregation studies can also be complicated by variable expressivity, reduced penetrance, nonpaternity, and the age of disease onset. As per ACMG/AMP criteria, co-segregation with disease in multiple affected family members in a gene

known to cause the disease provides only "Supporting" evidence. This can be upgraded if the variant has been reported to segregate with disease in multiple families of diverse ethnic backgrounds.

d. Follow-up on variants of uncertain significance

- Multigene panels often yield more VUSs compared to ES/GS. Laboratories may be more inclined to report every variant they identify on panels but are more selective with ES/GS.
- Missense, in-frame indel variants, and intronic (noncanonical) variants are more likely to be reported as VUSs than loss-of-protein function (LOF) variants, such as nonsense, frameshift, or canonical splice site variants.
- LOF variants, like those causing premature termination of translation (nonsense or frameshift variants) and canonical splice site variants, may be classified as VUSs if haploinsufficiency is not a known disease mechanism of the gene. The likelihood of a gene being LOF intolerant (or haploinsufficient) can be inferred from gnomAD scores, such as pLI (probability of being LoF intolerant) and LOEUF (LoF observed/expected upper bound fraction). The ClinGen Dosage Sensitivity Workgroup also publishes gene curations on the ClinGen website. LOF variants may also be classified as VUSs if they are located in the 3′ end of the gene (as resulting mRNA may escape nonsense-mediated decay or produce a truncated yet functional protein) or if the variant is found in an exon absent in the biologically relevant transcript. Please refer to ClinGen's updated recommendations on interpreting LOF variants.

Evidence that may reclassify a VUS includes:

- *Has the variant been reported in affected individuals?* If prevalence of the variant in affected individuals is significantly increased compared to controls, it is considered a Strong piece of evidence. However, for case-control studies of very rare variants that may not reach statistical significance, laboratories may downgrade the evidence from Strong to Moderate or Supporting.
- *Has the variant been reported in the most recent and diverse control databases?* The absence/rarity of a variant in control databases should be downgraded to Supporting evidence as per 2020 ClinGen recommendations.
- *Have any functional studies performed on the variant?* This could be the most informative evidence to reclassify a variant. Refer to ClinGen's guidelines on how to use functional evidence in variant interpretation for additional information.
- *Family studies* (see earlier section)
- *Location of the variant within the gene:* Determining that a missense variant is found in a mutational hotspot or in a critical functional domain without benign variation can suggest pathogenicity. For LOF variants, identifying downstream disease-causing LOFs can be used as evidence of pathogenicity.

- In silico *predictors* (for missense and splice variants only): Since 2022, ClinGen recommends using the score from a single tool (BayesDel, MutPred2, REVEL, or VEST4) to upgrade or downgrade a missense variant. In 2023, the ClinGen SVI Splicing Subgroup released recommendations on using prediction tools for splice variants.

e. Variants in genes of uncertain significance (GUS)

- As per the original ACMG/AMP publication, variants in genes not yet associated with disease should be classified as variants in "genes of uncertain significance" (GUS).
- If a variant in a GUS is found in your client, efforts should be undertaken to identify additional individuals with variants in the same gene. This may result in the creation of a cohort and the publication of a new gene–disease association, potentially resulting in the reclassification of the variant.
- Resources such as GeneMatcher, the Matchmaker Exchange, and the Deciphering Developmental Disorders (DDD) Study help connect with clinicians and researchers who have identified other individuals with variants in the same gene. Tools such as MyGene2 allow families to create profiles and connect.
- Setting up alerts on PubMed and OMIM is a useful way to stay updated on a gene of interest.

Case Study

Trio exome sequencing was ordered in 2019 on a 10-year-old male with developmental delays, hearing loss, autism, and macrocephaly and showed a *de novo* missense variant in the *RAC1* gene described as *RAC1* (NM_006908.3):c.190T>G; p.(Tyr64Asp). *RAC1* was recently linked to a developmental disorder with variable features, and missense variants were found to act through constitutive activation or a dominant-negative effect. At the time, the variant was classified as a VUS, as it had only been described in one individual to date, the gene–disease association was recent, and the disease mechanism was still being investigated.

The variant can now be reclassified to pathogenic based on evidence found in a new publication by Banka et al. (2022):

- **Other affected individuals with the same variant**: The publication includes four more individuals with the same variant as seen in our client.
- **Other relevant variants**: The paper also includes an individual with a different amino acid change at the same residue (p.Tyr64Cys).
- **Functional studies**: These are consistent with the variant having an activating effect by causing morphological changes in embryonic neurons, disorganization of axon fascicles in the embryonic CNS, and increased branching of sensory neurons.

- **Critical functional domain information**: The variant is found within a critical region known as Switch II, where several missense variants have been reported to be disease-associated. Activating missense variants in residues Gln61-Arg68 are associated with a developmental phenotype.
- *In silico* **predictors**: A REVEL score of 0.922 allows to upgrade the evidence of *in silico* predictors from Supporting to Moderate.

KEY POINT SUMMARY

- Guidelines of variant interpretation are regularly being revised. Therefore, the classification of a variant may change over time.
- Family studies, the presence of a variant in control or disease databases, functional studies, and other factors should be interpreted according to the latest guidelines to determine if a variant can be reclassified.
- Since there is no consensus on who is responsible for initiating a reanalysis or reinterpretation, it is advised to contact the clinical laboratory director or genetic counselor with questions about a specific variant.

Bibliography

ClinGen. https://clinicalgenome.org
ClinGen's Dosage Sensitivity Curations. https://search.clinicalgenome.org/kb/gene-dosage?page=1&size=25&search=
ClinGen's Sequence Variant Interpretation Working Group (SVI WG). https://clinicalgenome.org/working-groups/sequence-variant-interpretation/
ClinVar. https://www.ncbi.nlm.nih.gov/clinvar/
Deciphering Developmental Disorders (DDD) Study, DECIPHER. https://www.decipher genomics.org/ddd/overview
Franklin. https://franklin.genoox.com/
Genematcher. https://genematcher.org/
gnomAD. https://gnomad.broadinstitute.org/
Lift Over Tool. https://liftover.broadinstitute.org/
Matchmaker Exchange. https://www.matchmakerexchange.org/
MyGene2. https://mygene2.org/MyGene2/
OMIM. https://www.omim.org/
PubMed. https://pubmed.ncbi.nlm.nih.gov/
Variant Effect Predictor. http://grch37.ensembl.org/common/Tools/VEP?db=core; https://www.ncbi.nlm.nih.gov/clinvar/
Varsome. https://varsome.com/

Abou Tayoun AN et al. ClinGen Sequence Variant Interpretation Working Group (ClinGen SVI). Recommendations for interpreting the loss of function PVS1 ACMG/AMP variant criterion. *Hum Mutat*. 2018;39(11):1517–1524. https://doi.org/10.1002/humu.23626
Appelbaum PS et al. Is there a duty to reinterpret genetic data? The ethical dimensions. *Genet Med*. 2020;22(3):633–639. https://doi.org/10.1038/s41436-019-0679-7

Banka S et al. Activating RAC1 variants in the switch II region cause a developmental syndrome and alter neuronal morphology. *Brain*. 2022;145(12):4232–4245. https://doi.org/10.1093/brain/awac049

Boycott KM et al. Seven years since the launch of the Matchmaker Exchange: The evolution of genomic matchmaking. *Hum Mutat*. 2022;43(6):659–667. https://doi.org/10.1002/humu.24373

Brnich SE et al. On behalf of the Clinical Genome Resource Sequence Variant Interpretation Working Group. Recommendations for application of the functional evidence PS3/BS3 criterion using the ACMG/AMP sequence variant interpretation framework. *Genome Med*. 2020;12:3. https://doi.org/10.1186/s13073-019-0690-2

Clinical Genome Resource (ClinGen). *SVI Recommendation for Absence/Rarity (PM2) - Version 1.0*, Approved September 2020. https://clinicalgenome.org/site/assets/files/5182/pm2_-_svi_recommendation_-_approved_sept2020.pdf

Clinical Genome Resource (ClinGen). *SVI Recommendation for De Novo Criteria (PS2 & PM6) - Version 1.1*, Updated 2021. https://clinicalgenome.org/site/assets/files/3461/svi_proposal_for_de_novo_criteria_v1_1.pdf

Firth HV et al. DECIPHER: Database of Chromosomal Imbalance and Phenotype in Humans Using Ensembl Resources. *Am J Hum Genet*. 2009;84:524–533. https://doi.org/10.1016/j.ajhg.2009.03.010

Gudmundsson S et al. Variant interpretation using population databases: Lessons from gnomAD. *Hum Mutat*. 2022;43(8):1012–1030. https://doi.org/10.1002/humu.24309

Macklin S et al. Observed frequency and challenges of variant reclassification in a hereditary cancer clinic. *Genet Med*. 2018;20(3):346–350. https://doi.org/10.1038/gim.2017.207

Mersch J et al. Prevalence of variant reclassification following hereditary cancer genetic testing. *JAMA*. 2018;320(12):1266–1274. https://doi.org/10.1001/jama.2018.13152

Pejaver V et al. ClinGen Sequence Variant Interpretation Working Group. Calibration of computational tools for missense variant pathogenicity classification and ClinGen recommendations for PP3/BP4 criteria. *Am J Hum Genet*. 2022;109(12):2163–2177. https://doi.org/10.1016/j.ajhg.2022.10.013

Rehm HL et al. Medical Genome Initiative Steering Committee. The landscape of reported VUS in multi-gene panel and genomic testing: Time for a change. *Genet Med*. 2023;25(12):100947. https://doi.org/10.1016/j.gim.2023.100947

Reijnders MRF et al. RAC1 missense mutations in developmental disorders with diverse phenotypes. *Am J Hum Genet*. 2017;101(3):466–477. https://doi.org/10.1016/j.ajhg.2017.08.007

Richards S et al. ACMG Laboratory Quality Assurance Committee. Standards and guidelines for the interpretation of sequence variants: A joint consensus recommendation of the American College of Medical Genetics and Genomics and the Association for Molecular Pathology. *Genet Med*. 2015;17(5):405–424. https://doi.org/10.1038/gim.2015.30

Sobreira N et al. GeneMatcher: A matching tool for connecting investigators with an interest in the same gene. *Hum Mutat*. 2015;36(10):928–930. https://doi.org/10.1002/humu.22844

Walker LC et al. ClinGen Sequence Variant Interpretation Working Group. Using the ACMG/AMP framework to capture evidence related to predicted and observed impact on splicing: Recommendations from the ClinGen SVI Splicing Subgroup. *Am J Hum Genet*. 2023;110(7):1046–1067. https://doi.org/10.1016/j.ajhg.2023.06.002

2

The Role of Race, Ethnicity, and Ancestry in Genomic Testing

AISHWARYA ARJUNAN,
KATELYNN G. SAGASER, AND
SALLY A. RODRIGUEZ

Introduction

Despite a professional obligation to "do no harm," racism in medicine has long been pervasive, and we must dismantle and unlearn practices that contribute to gaps and disparities in care. Population descriptors such as **race**, **ethnicity**, and **ancestry** (REA) have been used by researchers to examine patterns of human genetic variation due to history, migration, and evolution. The general public, clinicians, and researchers alike tend to use the concepts of REA interchangeably, although they are not equivalent (Table 2.1). This practice has influenced many aspects of medical research and education, perpetuating racial discrimination in healthcare and negatively impacting all elements of medicine.

Although race and ethnicity are both social constructs, these personal descriptors have been used within medical practice to dictate the type of care an individual receives. While some of these incorporations were based on observed epidemiological data, many have failed to account for the underlying systemic structures and barriers that play a significant role in these health outcomes. **Social determinants of health (SDOH)** – conditions that affect a wide range of health, functioning, quality-of-life outcomes, and risk – also profoundly impact patient outcomes. SDOH encompasses economic stability, access to and quality of education and healthcare, and environmental and social context. When risk assessment tools and treatment guidelines incorporate race and ethnicity without accounting for SDOH, they risk perpetuating the belief that race alone predicts health outcomes. Clinicians should be able to identify that different population groups may have variation in disease prevalence or susceptibility, but we cannot allow race to be used as a shorthand for genetic predilection to health and well-being. This chapter will examine how we use race and ethnicity in the care that we provide and the research that we conduct so that we can dismantle these systems and practices.

DOI: 10.1201/9781003397847-2

Table 2.1 Definitions of Race, Ethnicity, and Ancestry per the National Academies of Sciences, Engineering, and Medicine

TERM	DEFINITION
Race	A sociopolitically constructed system for classifying and ranking human beings according to subjective beliefs about shared ancestry based on perceived innate biological similarities; the system varies globally
Ethnicity	A sociopolitically constructed system for classifying human beings according to claims of shared heritage often based on perceived cultural similarities (e.g., language, religion, beliefs); the system varies globally
Ancestry	A person's origin or descent, lineage, "roots," or heritage, including kinship

Challenges and Strategies

REA Data Collection

Within genetic medicine, a patient's self-reported ethnicity and/or race has historically been used to determine the genetic test offered and, thus, the comprehensiveness of the genetic evaluation provided. As part of genetic test selection, patients may be offered different panels depending on their race or ethnicity, a paradigm known as **race/ethnicity-based screening**. However, in order for race/ethnicity-based screening to be effective, patient racial and ethnic background information must be (1) able to be collected, (2) accurate, and (3) well studied within the medical literature so that allele frequency and disease incidence data are known. Yet in practice, these criteria are rarely met. Counselors should question whenever REA is used to dictate the care provided. Is there actually a need to ask a patient's ethnicity? For what purpose is the information being used? We must educate our cross-disciplinary colleagues about the impact to patient care when REA is used in clinical practice and advocate to change these practices.

Given that the field of medical genetics was birthed in an era when antimiscegenation laws were typical, many standard practices are no longer applicable, accurate, or equitable today. Despite a growing multiracial population, clinical guidelines are primarily based on the assumption of an individual having a single race or ethnicity, and genomic databases used to create guidelines are composed of data from primarily white individuals. A 276% increase in the multiracial populations was seen between 2010 and 2020. Additionally, 1 out of every 6 new marriages are between individuals of different ethnic backgrounds. Furthermore, 4 out of 10 Americans are unable to correctly identify the ancestry of all four of their grandparents, and 10% of individuals have a 50% or greater genetic ancestry different from what they self-report. Few medical management recommendations exist for individuals reporting multiracial ancestry, adoption, or uncertain ancestry, illustrating the manner in which race/ethnicity-based screening practices can leave patients behind. We must closely evaluate genetic testing paradigms and protocols for bias due to REA.

Lack of Diversity in Genomic Databases

Genomic research is dependent on the samples and data included in various international biobanks and databases. In order to provide equal benefit, these databases must be diverse. However, between 2009 and 2016, the proportion of data coming from individuals of European descent only decreased from 96% to 81% despite a more than 20-fold increase in the number of samples included. For reference, individuals of European descent made up 10% of the world population in 2016. The majority of the increase in the non-European proportion of samples came from individuals of Asian descent, with less than 5% of samples coming from people of African, Hispanic and Latin American, Pacific Islander, Arab and Middle Eastern, Indigenous, and Mixed ancestry *combined*. These significant disparities in data inevitably result in downstream negative effects and further exacerbate health inequities.

Genetic counselors play key roles across every area of genomic medicine and have a unique opportunity to impact genomic research. Those involved in research roles or projects should consider study design and recruitment strategies that maximize diversity and equity. REA data should be collected responsibly – including allowing patients or participants to self-identify their race or ethnicity, ensuring the REA terminology and categories are accurate, and allowing individuals to select multiple options or decline to self-identify. With increasing efforts across healthcare, the hope and goal is to diversify genomic databases. In the meantime, we should be mindful of the most immediate consequences of nondiverse databases: higher rates of variants of uncertain significance (VUS) for non-white patients and thus increased difficulty with genetic diagnoses and, where applicable, treatment decisions. These are not insignificant issues given the potential downstream effects of delayed treatments for various genetic conditions. Counselors in clinical settings should consider implementing protocols for ensuring appropriate follow-up for all patients with VUS results, especially those who would benefit from reclassification in regard to treatment, reproductive decision-making, and so on.

Bias in Guidelines and Practice in Genetics

The negative effects of REA-based guidelines can be seen in various areas within genomics. For example, in oncology, the 3-variant *BRCA1/2* founder mutation panel for individuals of Ashkenazi Jewish (AJ) descent was once a routine offering. However, an ethnicity-specific panel creates inequality given that AJ individuals could also have non-AJ ancestry and thus be at risk for other variants that would be missed. Furthermore, if screened for "eligibility" based on REA, individuals without known AJ ancestry may miss an opportunity for testing and be unaware of their increased cancer risk. Though not routine today in cancer genetics clinics, this 3-variant panel offering still exists and may be ordered by providers who may be unaware of the limitations. Despite a similar prevalence of pathogenic cancer susceptibility variants in Black and non-Hispanic white women, there are lower genetic testing rates among Black women with breast cancer. We must question what guidelines and biases are leading to the discrepancy in testing uptake given the significant downstream effects.

In the carrier screening space, screening guidelines for cystic fibrosis (CF) focused on a small panel of ~25 variants for nearly 20 years despite said panel having subpar detection rates outside of the non-Hispanic white and Ashkenazi Jewish populations and even after major technological advancements permitted screening on a much larger scale. The impact can be seen in patient outcomes: (1) non-white infants with CF are more likely to be older at diagnosis and have failure to thrive, (2) Black and Hispanic individuals with CF are underrepresented in clinical research and thus are less likely to benefit from precision medicine treatments targeting variants prevalent in European populations, and (3) Black and Hispanic individuals with CF have a two-fold increased risk of dying before the age of 18 years compared to white individuals with CF. Fortunately, in 2021, the American College of Medical Genetics (ACMG) issued updated guidelines on carrier screening acknowledging the need to eliminate REA-based recommendations, as they are "both inequitable and scientifically flawed." However, the American College of Obstetricians and Gynecologists (ACOG) reaffirmed its existing carrier screening guidelines in 2023, which still indicate that an ethnic-specific (as well as panethnic and expanded) carrier screening approach is acceptable. Given that most carrier screening continues to be facilitated by general OB/GYNs and reproductive endocrinologists, who often primarily follow ACOG guidelines, change may be slow.

Additional examples of bias exist within prenatal care that contribute to health disparities:

- A large retrospective study recently challenged the adjustment of maternal serum alpha fetoprotein screening results based on race, as no difference in values was observed between Black and non-Black pregnant patients after adjusting for maternal weight and gestational age.
- Cell-free DNA (cfDNA) screening for chromosomal aneuploidy is currently the most sensitive screening option during pregnancy. However, individuals with high body mass index (BMI) have a higher risk for a nonreportable result. This risk may be as high as ~25% due to the correlation between increasing BMI and reduced fetal fraction. As such, ACMG recommended an alternative to cfDNA for pregnant patients with "significant obesity." Notably, BMI was developed by an 1830s mathematician whose study included exclusively Western European men, making BMI unevenly applicable across populations.
- A study highlighted a lower fetal fraction in *HBB* carriers compared to non-carriers. Thus, as non-white individuals have a higher likelihood of *HBB* carrier status, they also potentially have a higher risk for test failure based on fetal fraction cutoffs.

The development and growing use of polygenic risk scores (PRS) is also a significant area of concern in regard to REA data within genomics. PRS algorithms are developed using data from genome-wide association studies and/or genomic databases, which are currently ~80% European and thus inherently biased. Until genomic databases accurately reflect global populations, the applicability of PRS models for non-white patients is debatable. If the use of PRS becomes commonplace for screening eligibility/coverage determination, health outcome disparities could worsen, as early or frequent screening in high-risk individuals is often the best way to prevent morbidity and mortality. The *possible* clinical utility of PRS is significant – identifying higher-risk individuals for prioritization in clinical assessments and health screenings could save countless lives – but its true potential cannot be known until the underlying data is reliable. Given that PRS models are already in use or in development across various specialties, including oncology, cardiology, and reproductive care, thinking about and addressing these issues soon is essential.

Real-World Case Study

In March 2024, direct-to-consumer genetic testing company 23andMe released three new PRS reports for subscription members – a breast cancer report (females only based on self-reported birth sex), a prostate cancer report (males only based on self-reported birth sex), and a colorectal cancer report. These reports were developed from 23andMe's proprietary research database, and with more than 15 million customers, 23andMe boasts one of the largest and most diverse genomic datasets in the world. The company acknowledged the limitations of the new PRS reports in an accompanying press release, noting that the colorectal cancer report is only available for customers of European and Latino/Hispanic descent, "as there is not yet enough data to provide a result for those of other ethnicities." Earlier in the same month, 23andMe announced the launch of the "Genetic Insights into Colorectal Cancer in the Black Community Study," recruiting individuals with a personal history of colorectal cancer, age 18 years and older with African ancestry and/or identifying as Black or African American. The company's press release went on to describe their hope of gathering sufficient data from this study to improve PRS and inform Black or African American individuals of their colorectal cancer risk. Establishing and maintaining trust with the Black/African American community is essential to the success of this study, as participation in research can be fraught with concerns about the use of genomic data. This example highlights the difficulties of launching new reports and tools that are equitable across all populations and how centuries of inequitable research fuel disparities in the availability and/or utility of risk-prediction tools.

The first step in bringing about meaningful change within genomic medicine is to acknowledge the backdrop of systemic racism that affects every aspect of healthcare within the United States. The solutions must be multifaceted: (1) question your assumptions and routine practices, (2) collect REA data responsibly, (3) be purposeful in genetic testing selections and offerings, and (4) advocate for change within professional organizations and from healthcare payors. Furthermore, as healthcare professionals show a "united front" focused on equitable care, we can push payors to update their coverage policies in order to make genetic testing more accessible. While centuries of harm cannot be undone overnight, good-faith efforts, humility, intentionality, and perseverance are crucial for making strides toward a more equitable society.

KEY POINT SUMMARY

- Race, ethnicity, and ancestry are three different population descriptors not to be used interchangeably, and their use in practice should be questioned and reexamined.
- The social construct of race must be disentangled from genetic ancestry, and the clinician's focus must be fixed on SDOH in a way that truly addresses health disparities.
- Genomic research is dependent on the samples and data included in various international biobanks and databases, and in order for studies to benefit all individuals equally, these databases must be diverse.
- Clinical guidelines that utilize REA to dictate the type of care that is provided or testing that is offered and available to patients need to be reexamined and rewritten.
- It is imperative to examine practices and unlearn behaviors that contribute to existing disparities.

Bibliography

ACOG Committee on Genetics. Committee opinion 486: Update on carrier screening for cystic fibrosis. *Obstet Gynecol*. 2011;117(4):1028–1031.

ACOG Committee on Genetics. Committee opinion 690: Carrier screening in the age of genomic medicine. *Obstet Gynecol*. 2017a;129:e35–e40.

ACOG Committee on Genetics. Committee opinion 691: Carrier screening for genetic conditions. *Obstet Gynecol*. 2017b;129(3):e41–e55.

Arjunan A et al. Addressing reproductive healthcare disparities through equitable carrier screening: Medical racism and genetic discrimination in United States' history highlights the needs for change in obstetrical genetics care. *Societies*. 2022;12:33. https://doi.org/10.3390/soc12020033

Australian Broadcasting Corporation. *The Really Old, Racist and Non-Medical Origins of the BMI*, 2022. www.abc.net.au/news/2022-01-02/the-problem-with-the-body-mass-index-bmi/100728416

Burns RN et al. Reconsidering race adjustment in prenatal alpha-fetoprotein screening. *Obstet Gynecol*. 2023;141(3):438–444. Erratum in: *Obstet Gynecol*. 2023;141(6):1229.

Condit C et al. Attitudinal barriers to delivery of race-targeted pharmacogenomics among informed lay persons. *Genet Med*. 2003;5:385–392.

Crandall BF et al. Alpha-fetoprotein concentrations in maternal serum: Relation to race and body weight. *Clin Chem*. 1983;29(3):531–533.

Cystic Fibrosis Foundation. *CF Foundation Seeks Input from Communities of Color [Internet]*, 2020. www.cff.org/news/2020–11/cf-foundation-seeks-input-communities-color

Domchek SM et al. Comparison of the prevalence of pathogenic variants in cancer susceptibility genes in black women and non-Hispanic white women with breast cancer in the United States. *JAMA Oncol.* 2021;7(7):1045–1050.

Gregg AR et al. Noninvasive prenatal screening for fetal aneuploidy, 2016 update: A position statement of the American College of Medical Genetics and Genomics. *Genet Med.* 2016;18(10):1056–1065.

Hunt LM et al. Genes, race, and culture in clinical care: Racial profiling in the management of chronic illness. *Med Anthropol Q.* 2013;27:253–271.

Kaseniit KE et al. Genetic ancestry analysis on >93,000 individuals undergoing expanded carrier screening reveals limitations of ethnicity-based medical guidelines. *Genet Med.* 2020;22:1694–1702.

Landry LG et al. Lack of diversity in genomic databases is a barrier to translating precision medicine research into practice. *Health Aff (Millwood).* 2018;37(5):780–785.

Livingston G. *Brown A. Pew Research Center: Intermarriage in the U.S. 50 Years after Loving v. Virginia.* www.pewresearch.org/social-trends/2017/05/18/intermarriage-in-the-u-s -50-years-after-loving-v-virginia/

Muzzey D et al. Noninvasive prenatal screening for patients with high body mass index: Evaluating the impact of a customized whole genome sequencing workflow on sensitivity and residual risk. *Prenat Diagn.* 2020;40(3):333–341.

National Academies of Sciences, Engineering, and Medicine. *Advancing Antiracism, Diversity, Equity, and Inclusion in STEMM Organizations: Beyond Broadening Participation.* National Academies Press, 2023. https://doi.org/10.17226/26902

Popejoy A, Fullerton S. Genomics is failing on diversity. *Nature.* 2016;538:161–164. https://doi .org/10.1038/538161a

Population Reference Bureau. *2016 World Population Data Sheet [Internet].* https://www.prb.org/ resources/2016-world-population-data-sheet/

Putra M et al. The impact of HBB-related hemoglobinopathies carrier status on fetal fraction in noninvasive prenatal screening. *Prenat Diagn.* 2022;42(4):524–529.

Sirugo G et al. The missing diversity in human genetic studies. *Cell.* 2019;177(1):26–31. Erratum in: *Cell.* 2019;177(4):1080.

U.S. Census Bureau. *Improved Race and Ethnicity Measures Reveal U.S. Population is Much More Multiracial [Internet]*, 2021. https://www.census.gov/library/stories/2021/08/improved- race-ethnicity-measures-reveal-united-states-population-much-more-multiracial.html

3

RESEARCH GENETIC TESTING

NATALIE C. LIPPA

Introduction

Clinical and research genetic testing have always been interconnected as newly discovered genetic findings are eventually integrated into clinical testing. Prior to the advent of next-generation sequencing (NGS), the identification of novel genetic syndromes was often done through familial studies via linkage studies. In practice, the line between research and clinical testing cannot always be clearly defined. However, it is good practice to confirm all research findings in a clinical laboratory.

The goal of the Clinical Laboratory Improvement Amendments (CLIA) Program is to ensure quality laboratory testing and that clinical laboratories meet specific standards. CLIA-certified laboratories are subject to stringent regulation from government and states. For instance, CLIA-certified laboratories are subject to inspections and analytic validity testing. For these reasons, it is important to confirm research findings in a CLIA-certified laboratory. In some cases, research findings cannot be confirmed in a CLIA-certified laboratory because no such laboratory offered testing of the newly discovered gene. In other cases, the research deployed a new genomic technology that was not available in a CLIA-certified laboratory. Indeed, this author has experienced cases in which a research finding was included in a physician's clinic note, but the finding was not (nor could not be) confirmed in a CLIA-certified laboratory.

Large-scale research studies, such as the *All of Us*, will routinely be returning genomic results to participants. The goal is to directly impact clinical care through genetic testing, and results include ACMG secondary as well as pharmacogenomic findings. However, results from the *All of Us* study may not be confirmed in a CLIA-certified laboratory prior to being returned to the research subject. This chapter will describe specific scenarios that a genetic counselor may encounter in regard to research genetic testing.

Challenges and Strategies

Counseling Clients with Research Genetic Testing Results

As large-scale research studies are deployed across the country, a clinical genetic counselor will likely encounter a client that arrives to their clinic with a genetic test

DOI: 10.1201/9781003397847-3

report from a research study. Given the more stringent oversight of CLIA-certified laboratories, confirmation of the finding in the CLIA space is recommended. For example, a sample swap may be more likely to occur in a research lab because testing is often completed on deidentified samples, whereas CLIA laboratories have well established processes to maintain chain of custody of the sample.

When preparing for the client's appointment, it is important to gather documents that describe the research study. Knowing why the client enrolled in the study and what eligibility criteria were met would also be worth exploring. If possible, obtaining the research notes about why a genomic variant was reported could also help you prepare for the visit. Medical records related to the research finding from outside institutions can also be helpful. For instance, if the client has a genetic finding in a cardiomyopathy gene, notes and evaluations from their cardiologist would also be useful for variant interpretation.

Starting the session by understanding the client's motivation to enroll in the research study is a good way to build rapport and understand their knowledge of the research finding. This should be followed by a medical and family history. If possible, it would be ideal if this information could be obtained prior to the actual session to help prepare for the visit. Additionally, the client may have other clinical features that may warrant different clinical genetic testing or referrals.

Describe this genomic finding and the known gene–disease associations. Variant level details can also be shared with the client. Specific information related to how the research finding either explains their personal history of disease or could impact their care. For instance, this could include details related to pharmacogenetic findings and any current or future medications.

It is possible that the client does not know specific differences between research and clinical testing. This conversation should be put into context depending on the research design and eligibility requirements. Dialogue about the need for CLIA confirmation is also essential to communicate to the client. A research result must be confirmed before any treatment/management changes are made. Acting on a research finding could result in unnecessary evaluations and referrals.

A discussion about GINA and other insurance discrimination is also important, especially for asymptomatic individuals.

The cost of the genetic test should also be addressed because it is possible that insurance companies may not cover the price of testing. Therefore, the CLIA confirmation process may result in a out-of-pocket expense for the client, and depending on the research consent process, it is imaginable that the client may not have been aware of the additional expenses that could be incurred prior to enrolling in the research study.

Choosing a CLIA-Certified Laboratory

If the client decides to continue with genetic testing, it is important to send to a CLIA-certified laboratory if practicing within the United States.

CLIA regulates human specimen laboratories to ensure accurate and reliable results. Please note that in some cases, the research result may already have been confirmed in a CLIA laboratory, at which point, it may not be necessary to redo the genetic testing.

In some states, such as in New York, a laboratory also needs to have an approval/license from that state. In some cases, you can request a waiver of this requirement.

The CLIA confirmation process involves sending a new identified sample to a CLIA-certified lab. Using a deidentified sample may not be acceptable by a clinical laboratory, as the chain of custody has been broken.

For some genetic findings, the identification of a CLIA laboratory that can perform appropriate testing may be straightforward and as simple as ordering a single site test. However, in other situations, it may be difficult to order the genetic test. For instance, special assays are required to identify certain pharmacogenetic findings, and there are limited laboratories that offer such testing. Testing for some of the variants may more easily (and more affordably) be done by ordering another gene panel (ensuring that the research variant is on the panel) from a CLIA laboratory. The Genetic Testing Registry website can help identify a laboratory that may analyze the gene of interest. It is recommended to contact the laboratory to confirm that it can identify and report the variant of interest given limitations of genetic tests (i.e., intronic variants, deletions/duplications).

Finally, there may be scenarios in which genetic technology has advanced more rapidly in the research space than in the clinical genetic realm. In these situations, a discussion with the research team may be warranted. The research team may have options for you and the family in regard to clinical genetic testing or may be able to advise on standard-of-care genetic tests that can be ordered to replicate the research findings (i.e., an optical mapping finding that can be seen on microarray). They might also be able to provide a more detailed account of the genetic diagnosis identified in the research. Requesting the research team share their published findings (once available) can also be useful to the client.

Outdated Research Genetic Report Findings

There are a few things to consider if a client brings in a genetic report from a research study that has not been completed in recent years. The first is that the genetic notations and nomenclature might be out of date due to using older genomic builds. In some cases, sending the report to the CLIA lab can help. Alternatively, full sequencing of the gene may be required.

The second consideration is related to the quality of the research and whether the tools used previously are still valid. For instance, one can imagine single gene studies in which a "mutation" was identified that is now clearly considered benign. Depending on family history and developed client phenotype, a more thorough genetic investigation could be helpful such as with exome or genome.

Contributing to a Genetic Research Study Design

There are many aspects in which a genetic counselor can contribute to the design of a genetic research study. The following items of consideration will help organize your thoughts as you work to understand the research design. Additionally, this will help the research team communicate the study clearly to research subjects in the IRB-approved consent form.

   a. *What is the research question?*
      i. This is one of the most important questions you should consider. What question do you and the researchers hope to answer? For example, does the research aim to elucidate the genetic contribution to disease or explore return of results and assess the clinical utility and psychosocial impact of the results?
   b. *What type of genetic testing will the study complete?*
      i. Genetic and genomic technology have advanced relatively quickly, yet our understanding of genetic variation has not advanced at the same speed.
      ii. Here, it is also important to define variant classification and variant filtering. How will this be completed? In some cases, this may be part of the research process to understand the best way to filter variants to determine genotype–phenotype relationships.
      iii. For polygenic risks scores, how will score be validated? Is validation necessary?
      iv. Where will the genetic testing be done – in a CLIA or research laboratory?
   c. *What results will be returned?*
      i. Will the team report pathogenic or likely pathogenic variants?
      ii. Consider when you would report out VUS findings. For instance, would you only report there when there is a strong phenotypic overlap?
      iii. For polygenic risks scores, what is the threshold to report? Is there a threshold?
   d. *Communication of results*
      i. Will results be returned to participants? How will results be returned? Many research study personnel call the subject and then follow-up with a letter and/or email.
      ii. Will the study team return non-CLIA-confirmed results? In some cases, the study may pay for a separate CLIA confirmation, but another sample may be needed.
      iii. Who will return the results?
      iv. Will the results be automatically uploaded to the electronic medical record? Or will this be done only after the CLIA confirmation process?
      v. Will study personnel be available to answer questions?
      vi. Do you have referral sites in case a finding needs follow-up (in the case of ACMG secondary findings)?

Case Study

A 75-year-old male client was recently admitted to the hospital for right facial droop and dysarthria. He was found to have had a stroke and was prescribed clopidogrel at discharge, a "blood thinner" commonly prescribed to prevent strokes. A few weeks after being discharged, he received an email describing the results from a genomic research study. The non-CLIA-certified research results indicated that he was a *CYP2C19* intermediate metabolizer (IM). *CYP2C19* is a "metabolizer" gene, and variants in this gene affect drug metabolism. As the genetic counselor researched this pharmacogenetic finding, she discovered that clopidogrel is not as effective in intermediate metabolizers.

A thorough family history taken during the session was not suggestive of a strong family history of a genetic disease. Based on medical history or family history, there was no other clinical genetic testing that would be warranted. The client recalled being enrolled in the study and that this was an "all comer" study. He did not have a particular phenotype that prompted enrollment. Additionally, he understood that this finding was part of the pharmacogenomic panel included in the research. As the session continued, it was clear that the client did not understand the reasoning for repeating the test in a CLIA laboratory. Once the risk of a sample swap was described, the client finally recognized the value of repeating the test.

The confirmation of *CYP2C19* genotype proved trickier than expected. One lab offered the testing for a cost of $500. The client's insurance would not cover the genetic testing since pharmacogenetic testing is not part of routine medical care. A commercial panel is available that includes the analysis of this genotype but also includes other findings, such as cardiogenetic genes and hereditary cancer genes. This panel was less expensive ($300), but insurance would still not cover the cost of this test. As the two options for testing were described, the client, understandably, did not want to further uncover risks for other conditions at this time. On the other hand, the single-site testing was more expensive, and the medical bills were already adding up after his recent hospitalization.

In the end, the client decided to pay a higher amount for the single-site testing. The research results were confirmed in the CLIA laboratory. The client was switched to a different medication through his neurologist given these findings.

KEY POINT SUMMARY

- Clearly communicate to families the differences between research and clinical testing.
- Understand that research subjects may not remember the research study details.
- If possible, CLIA confirm all research genetic testing results.

- Understand the research genetic testing process and why the study team deemed the finding to be reportable.
- Consider if a more thorough genetic investigation is warranted.

Bibliography

All of Us Research Program. *Program Overview [Internet]*. https://allofus.nih.gov/about/program-overview

Centers for Disease Control and Prevention. *Clinical Laboratory Improvement Amendments (CLIA) [Internet]*. www.cdc.gov/clia/about.html

Wadsworth Center. *Clinical Laboratory Evaluation Program (CLEP) – Test Approval [Internet]*. www.wadsworth.org/regulatory/clep/clinical-labs/obtain-permit/test-approval

4

CHALLENGING THE NORM OF NONDIRECTIVE COUNSELING

ERICA SPIEGEL

Introduction

Nondirectiveness has been a core tenet of genetic counseling since the birth of the profession, inspired by Carl Rogers's client-centered, empathic therapeutic model and adopted by the first Sarah Lawrence genetic counseling class. The aim of this counseling approach is to support clients in making decisions based on their beliefs, values, personal circumstances, and goals without influencing them toward a *specific* decision. The fundamental assumption is that the client is the expert in their own life. Nondirectiveness has been defined in various ways and holds diverse interpretations by genetic practitioners. It has historically been most practiced in reproductive genetic counseling because decision-making conversations are prevalent and can be emotionally, politically, and philosophically weighted.

Nondirectiveness in practice has been most commonly interpreted as providing balanced, value-neutral information and avoiding prescriptive medical advice or recommendations to clients. It is rooted in a desire to distance clinical genetics from past associations with eugenics and to honor the guiding professional principles of client self-directedness and empowerment. While well intentioned, the day-to-day practice of nondirectiveness can be challenging and, at its least effective, may lead to adverse effects or misguided care. Recent and ongoing genetic counseling conversations invoke consideration of a new perspective on nondirectiveness and question its place in the modern practice of genetic counseling.

Challenges and Strategies

Nondirectiveness May Inhibit or Interrupt Positive Relationship–Building with the Client

Clients very often arrive at genetic counseling without an understanding that the training and practice of genetic counselors is unique from that of physicians and other healthcare professionals. Clients may expect that communication within genetic counseling will follow traditional models of provider–client communication in which the provider offers medical recommendations, advice, and direction based on client history, test results, and examination, as well as best practices. As such, a client may be

DOI: 10.1201/9781003397847-4

disoriented by a medical visit that follows a different pattern, especially if an explanation of what to expect is not provided up front. Communication in which the client is made the sole decision-maker for important and sometimes emotional decisions can be anxiety inducing, overwhelming, or even frustrating if they anticipate receiving clear guidance and direct recommendations from their healthcare provider. At worst, a client who feels distressed or abandoned by the counselor may experience a reduction in their capacity to arrive at a decision or to develop a trusting relationship with the counselor, thus having the exact opposite effect of the one intended by genetic counseling.

Relatedly, the emphasis on individual autonomy in the Western model of nondirective counseling does not necessarily translate to the multicultural and diverse client population in the United States who may have less individualistic or more communal and family-oriented styles for medical decision-making or who may look for more directive-type guidance from medical experts.

As genetic information becomes more available *and* more complex, clients may feel more need or desire for recommendations from genetic providers who understand the nuances, risks, and benefits of potential genetic test results. In a study by Sullivan et al., only 13% of prospective parents hypothetically being offered whole-genome noninvasive prenatal screening (NIPS) wanted to make an independent decision about testing, whereas the majority wanted a clear recommendation from their provider or preferred joint decision-making.

Nondirectiveness Is Difficult to Implement in Practice and Easily Misunderstood by Practitioners

Challenges in rendering the *idea* of nondirectiveness into actual *practice* within clinical genetic counseling encounters abound. Nondirectiveness has been said to lack an "operational definition" (Elwyn) and may result in "hypervigilant non-interference" (Schupmann et al. 2020). Nondirectiveness by its nature is the absence of verbal or nonverbal communication to influence a client's behavior. It was intended to be an *active* strategy supported by counseling skills to encourage a client's autonomy and sense of competence. However, if nondirectiveness leads genetic counselors to shy away from select client-initiated topics (e.g., directly answering the question "What would you do?"), the counselor needs counterapproaches to address the client's questions (e.g., exploring what is behind the question or giving examples of what some clients do). In its most stringent application, nondirectiveness can result in the counselor taking a passive and distanced approach due to fear of being overly influential. Possession of other counseling models with skilled communication techniques is called for. Without these, genetic counselors may struggle to uphold a nondirective approach while still being attentive to the needs of a client seeking shared decision-making.

It has also been argued that nondirectiveness is not truly attainable. Weil (2003) defined four types of directiveness that are likely unavoidable. Two of those relevant to the individual genetic counselor are (1) inadvertent directiveness, in which the genetic counselor's values are apparent despite efforts to stay neutral and appear as such, and (2) inevitable directiveness, in which the genetic counselor's choice about the information they provide and their approach to counseling sends a message about their attitudes or values. A study of prenatal clients having diagnostic procedures showed that the uptake of fetal microarray varied significantly by genetic counselor even when controlling for other variables. This led the authors to conclude that genetic counselor preferences may have impacted client decisions. Genetic counselors will differ in the way they frame risk and present benefits, allocate time spent on each topic, and vary in word choice and nonverbal communication. Not surprisingly, genetic counselors' own biases and preferences can inevitably show through to the client.

Advances in Genomic Medicine and Existence of Best-Practice Guidelines Have Changed the Genetic Counseling Landscape

Nondirectiveness was born as the central tenet to genetic counseling when the field existed within only prenatal and pediatric genetics and decades before the existence of precision genomic medicine. Counseling was primarily based on pedigree interpretation, aneuploidy detection, and discussions of termination or continuation of pregnancy. In the 20th and early 21st centuries, preventative healthcare and management decisions based on genetic information were particularly limited by genetic knowledge and scarce testing options. Nondirectiveness remains a unanimous guiding principle today when delivering a *prenatal* diagnosis. "Nondirective" during prenatal results disclosure is an umbrella term that encourages neutrality, a nonjudgmental stance, and relaying balanced information. Counseling about a fetal diagnosis of Down syndrome, for example, involves highly personal decision-making about family building. Follow-up actions are not typically tied to a medical benefit or risk. The client's decision, guided by their values and goals rather than medical actionability, calls for equipoise.

As the role of genetics in other areas of health has grown, genetic counselors have become an increasing, sometimes routine presence in oncology, cardiology, neurology, and other subspecialties. These clients are often weighing treatment and management options in parallel with genetic counseling, and management may be informed by genetic results. A genetic diagnosis or a specific genotype–phenotype association could warrant changes to clinical care or uptake of specific health-promoting behaviors. When there is proven benefit to particular surveillance or treatment methods, a nondirective approach and clinical neutrality may not be in the client's best interest. The genetic counselor must weigh the ethical principle of client autonomy against those of beneficence and nonmaleficence and decide if a directional counseling approach is appropriate. In addition, the complex tasks that are now a routine part of genetic counseling may call for more than a purely nondirective approach. The counselor's expertise and communication skills ensure a client understands why they are being offered genetic testing, the decisions that are involved in consenting, and the possible impact of various test results. Clients may request counselor input in consent and testing decisions. Numerous evidence-based practice guidelines (American College of Medical Genetics, American College of Obstetrics and Gynecology, NCCN, etc.) on the appropriateness of genetic testing and follow-up best practices now exist. The genetic counselor thus has access to objective clinical recommendations that can be relayed to the client while concurrently evaluating their preferences and beliefs.

Strategies   There are both practical strategies and counseling techniques that can be implemented to address the challenges with nondirectiveness described here.

- Genetic counselor peer supervision groups, individual supervision or mentorship by a senior clinician, and continued education with attention to counseling skills are some ways that we can engage in reflective self-evaluation and ongoing learning and growth. In particular, peer supervision or "process" groups can provide genetic counselors a regularly scheduled time and supportive space to review challenging cases, to examine their approach and potential bias or assumptions, and to experiment with ideas and styles that are outside of the counselor's usual repertoire.

- Genetic counselors can explain the counseling process and role of the counselor during contracting to promote an understanding that they are there to provide information, share any relevant guidelines, learn about the client as a unique individual, and work in partnership to facilitate any decision-making that may be asked of them.

- Genetic counselors should remain up to date with practice guidelines and standard of care for their subspecialty. This knowledge can be shared with clients during the educational component of sessions to allow for fully informed decision-making. Client feelings and concerns around how genetic information would or wouldn't impact them or their family should be addressed. In cases in which there is a clear medical benefit to genetic testing in guiding medical management, prompting preventative measures, or allowing for familial cascade testing, a persuasive style of genetic counseling using motivational interviewing (MI) can be considered. MI and its application specifically to genetic counseling encounters are well described by Rescinow et al. and Ash. MI promotes directional (as opposed to directive) counseling. Shared decision-making (SDM) and the reciprocal engagement model (REM) of counseling are aligned with nondirective, client-centered genetic counseling. The REM was created specifically by genetic counselors for genetic counselors and includes specific strategies to meet goals. Both models underscore the importance of integrating teaching and counseling skills because neither teaching or counseling alone is sufficient. They recognize the value of relaying accurate information, presenting uncertainties and probabilities, and evaluating the client's emotions, beliefs, and core values. SDM stresses a two-way exchange and, refreshingly, builds in an expectation that the client and counselor will participate in joint decision-making, especially when there is a proven medical benefit of one course of action. Ultimately, the client's autonomy is respected and supported by the counselor. An update to the REM proposed by Biesecker acknowledges that challenging a patient's decision may be beneficial at times. For example, challenging may be appropriate if a clinically unaffected client declines cardiac follow-up despite having a pathogenic variant in *MYH7* (associated with hypertrophic cardiomyopathy).

In the long term, there should be continued efforts by the genetic counseling community and graduate programs to reduce attachment to nondirectiveness as a ruling principle because of the frequent misunderstanding of its application. A focus on training genetic counselors with active and varied counseling techniques that can be used to suit various scenarios would benefit counselors and clients. The goal should be to create a workforce of genetic counselors with flexibility, client responsiveness, and agility. Bringing a diverse counseling toolbox to each visit supports this mission.

Case Study

Marissa is a 36-year-old client, currently 10 weeks pregnant. Her first pregnancy resulted in a miscarriage at 10 weeks and was later found to have trisomy 18. She and her partner used *in vitro* fertilization (IVF) to conceive the current pregnancy after several months of trying unsuccessfully. Preimplantation genetic testing for aneuploidy (PGT-A) was normal. She was referred to discuss screening and diagnostic testing options and risks for a genetic condition based on history, prior results, and maternal age. During contracting, the genetic counselor (GC) asks how she has been feeling in the pregnancy. Marissa shares that she lies awake at night worrying about the risks for miscarriage and genetic issues. She is eager to get beyond 10 weeks and imagines feeling less anxious afterward. The GC responds empathically by validating her concern and normalizing the anxiety in a pregnancy after a miscarriage.

The GC reassures Marissa that PGT-A screened the embryo for trisomy 18 as well as other aneuploidies that increase in frequency with maternal age. The chance for this pregnancy to have aneuploidy is significantly reduced from the risk conferred by her age and obstetrical history. Her GC shares the guidance from ACOG that screening or diagnostic testing be offered in a pregnancy following PGT but assures her that she ultimately gets to decide if she wishes to pursue any testing. The GC describes the options of noninvasive prenatal screening, CVS, and amniocentesis, including their benefits, risks, and limitations.

Marissa would like to have diagnostic certainty but is nervous about the risk of miscarriage given her history. The GC empathizes that deciding between tests can be a tough decision and invites her to talk more about her concerns and priorities. She asks Marissa questions to better understand her thoughts and to increase Marissa's self-awareness of the most important factors contributing to her decision. The GC poses the following questions:

- What would it feel like for you to not have definitive results? If your blood work were normal, would this feel like sufficient information to be comfortable during the pregnancy?
- What is the risk you want to avoid the most?
- If you choose a screening test and it returns with a high-risk result, would this be useful to decide on confirmatory diagnostic testing?
- Would an abnormal test result from a diagnostic procedure impact your plans for the pregnancy?

Marissa shares that her biggest concern is the risk of miscarriage from a procedure, a devastating possible outcome. She doesn't feel that the gains from a diagnostic procedure warrant the risk. The genetic counselor summarizes what she heard and asks Marissa to correct any misunderstandings. She then explains that NIPS is the test that most aligns with her goals and expresses support for this selection. Marissa agrees and expresses relief with her decision.

KEY POINT SUMMARY

- Conversations around the utility and confines of nondirectiveness create an opportunity to reimagine its role in 21st-century clinical encounters.
- The principal challenges with nondirectiveness are difficulty in its successful implementation, the potential to disrupt budding counselor–client relationships, and developments in genomic medicine that can demand a more directional counseling style.
- Various strategies exist to address these challenges; these strategies should be mindful of balancing client autonomy with beneficence.
- The genetic counselor's intention to engage in shared decision-making and what this involves should be clearly communicated to clients at the start to reduce misunderstandings.
- Possession and utilization of counseling models beyond nondirectiveness is necessary. A combination of different techniques may be most effective even within a single counseling session.
- The genetic counseling community and training programs should consider de-emphasizing nondirectiveness as the core tenet of the field. Shifting the focus to engaged counseling strategies, such as those proposed by SDM and REM (among others), would increase the adaptability of genetic counselors and, in turn, benefit their clients.

Bibliography

American College of Obstetrics and Gynecology. Practice bulletin 226: Screening for fetal chromosomal abnormalities. *Obstet Gynecol*. 2020;136(4):859–867.

Ash E. Motivational interviewing in the reciprocal engagement model of genetic counseling: A method overview and case illustration. *J Genet Couns*. 2016;26(2):300–311.

Biesecker B. Genetic counseling and the central tenets of practice. *Cold Spring Harb Perspect Med*. 2019;10(3).

Eichinger J et al. 'It's a nightmare': Informed consent in paediatric genome-wide sequencing. A qualitative expert interview study from Germany and Switzerland. *Eur J Hum Genet*. 2023;31(12):1398–1406.

Elwyn G. Shared decision making and non-directiveness in genetic counselling. *J Med Genet*. 2000;37(2):135–138.

Kennedy AL. Supervision for practicing genetic counselors: An overview of models. *J Genet Couns*. 2000;9(5):379–390.

Kessler S. Psychological aspects of genetic counseling. VII. Thoughts on directiveness. *J Genet Couns*. 1992;1(1):9–17.

Resnicow K et al. Motivational interviewing for genetic counseling: A unified framework for persuasive and equipoise conversations. *J Genet Couns*. 2022;31(5):1020–1031.

Schupmann W et al. Re-examining the ethics of genetic counselling in the genomic era. *J Bioeth Inq*. 2020;17(3):325–335.

Sheets KB et al. Practice guidelines for communicating a prenatal or postnatal diagnosis of Down syndrome: Recommendations of the National Society of Genetic Counselors. *J Genet Couns*. 2011;20(5):432–441.

Sullivan HK et al. Noninvasive prenatal whole genome sequencing. *Obstet Gynecol*. 2019;133(3):525–532.

Swanson K et al. Disparities in the acceptance of chromosomal microarray at the time of prenatal genetic diagnosis. *Prenat Diagn*. 2022;42(5):611–616.

Veach PM et al. Coming full circle: A reciprocal-engagement model of genetic counseling practice. *J Genet Couns*. 2007;16(6):713–728.

Weil J. Psychosocial genetic counseling in the post-nondirective era: A point of view. *J Genet Couns*. 2003;12(3):199–211.

Weil J et al. The relationship of nondirectiveness to genetic counseling: Report of a workshop at the 2003 NSGC Annual Education Conference. *J Genet Couns*. 2006;15(2):85–93.

5

Loss and Grief in the Era of Genomic Medicine

AMANDA L. BERGNER

Introduction

Loss, the absence of something to which we were once attached, is a ubiquitous human experience. The widespread integration of genomics into healthcare can precipitate losses for our clients, including receipt of life-threatening or life-limiting diagnoses, lack of treatment or actionability following diagnostic results, uncertainty about the significance of genomic findings, misattributed family relationships, unanticipated (secondary) findings, ultra-rare diagnoses without communities of support, or the absence of a diagnosis even after intensive genomic investigation. To add complexity, genomic information often arrives during periods that are already emotionally intense, including pregnancy (fetal sequencing), acute illness (rapid inpatient sequencing), and death (sequencing of stillbirths, genomic autopsies, post-mortem testing). A normative response to loss is grief – the totality of emotional, cognitive, physical, behavioral, and spiritual experiences that occur as a person's interior and exterior life adjust to the loss.

While attending to loss and grief has always been part of the work of genetic counselors, the past 50 years have brought transformational changes in how loss and grief are understood. One of the first and still most widely recognized grief theories was the Kübler-Ross model, which outlined five stages of grief: denial, anger, bargaining, depression, and acceptance. Several other stage/phase models were introduced in the following years. While bringing order to a complex process, these early theories do not fully capture the complexity and diversity of the grieving experience. There has also been movement away from the idea that successful grieving involves severing ties (closure); rather, it requires continuing bonds that are conscious, dynamic, and changing. As well, the potential for posttraumatic growth and reconstructing meaning following loss is better understood. Loss and grief are often intense and disruptive, and they have the potential to result in psychoemotional growth, improved self-efficacy, and increased resilience. Our role as genetic counselors is to provide compassionate support to clients as they engage their grief while also facilitating their loss adaptation to relieve suffering and maximize the development of new capacities.

DOI: 10.1201/9781003397847-5

Challenges and Strategies

Recognizing Engagement with Client Loss and Grief as Key to the Work of Genetic Counselors

A necessary starting point is conceptualizing loss and grief as central to our work. No matter the clinical setting, we are in close contact with core aspects of human identity – health, parenting, (dis)ability, family, sexuality, work, and community. Our clients develop deep attachments within these aspects that make them who they are. When attachments are threatened or shifted, loss occurs. Common experiences are loss of security, control, physical and/or cognitive ability, certainty, employment, anticipated future, and relationships. Subsequent grief responses occur as our clients' lives and psyches reorganize to accommodate these changes. This period of vulnerability offers opportunity, as within this struggle lies the potential for significant personal growth. Facilitating client understanding, coping, and adaptation through these times reflects the psychotherapeutic potential of genetic counseling to improve client outcomes.

A note – while there are numerous challenges in this aspect of our work, this first is the most important to overcome because it can be particularly detrimental in the setting of providing fieldwork supervision for genetic counseling students. Practitioners may not only fail to model this central component of practice but may also message to developing counselors that they, too, should not engage clients in this way. Research demonstrates that perceived adequacy of training is by far the strongest predictor of practitioner comfort with grief, so it is central to educating future generations of genetic counselors that we engage this aspect of our own practice.

Becoming Comfortable with Loss and Grief

If loss and grief make you uncomfortable, you are not alone. A significant proportion of clinical genetics providers report lack of comfort in the presence of grief and loss even after repeated exposure through their work. This is an important challenge to address because the same providers report significantly higher clinician distress scores, making burnout more likely.

Consider inviting in experiences of loss and grief, beginning with your own. Helpful exercises can include creating a loss timeline, exploring loss inventories/worksheets, body awareness around sensations of grief, guided grief meditations, journaling about loss and grief (try the feelings wheel to expand your emotion-based vocabulary), or pursuing individual work with a therapist. Notice thoughts, feelings, and sensations that you want to move away from or ways in which you resist being fully present. These are clues to experiences you may move away from with your clients when counseling as well. It is possible that areas of unprocessed personal grief will be discovered that, once addressed, will expand your capacity to be present to your clients.

You can also engage the loss and grief of others through books, podcasts, movies, or other narratives. Try naming the losses people have experienced – both the initial (primary) loss and any downstream (secondary) losses. Practice naming feelings, both yours and those you observe in the narratives. You can also begin to notice how you feel after having engaged others' grief and explore further your capacity for bound-aried caring, where you are able to be present with another person's emotions while remaining grounded in yourself. As you invite it in, loss and grief can become more familiar and less uncomfortable.

Recognizing Client Loss and Grief

A good place to start can be case preparation. Based on what you know about the client, their life stage, and the reason for the visit, what loss(es) might they be expe-riencing? Not all sources of loss can be identified in advance of a session. Some will arise unexpectedly during sessions, which requires a general readiness. Familiarizing yourself with common losses in genetic/genomic medicine and those that arise most often for the client population you work with can be helpful.

Developing an understanding of the range of possible grief responses and those that are more common can improve your ability to recognize them. Common grief manifestations include:

- *Affective/feelings* – Shock, sadness, anger, guilt, helplessness, apathy, yearning/longing, anxiety, fear
- *Cognitive/thoughts* – Disbelief, confusion, overwhelm, preoccupation, halluci-nations, vivid dreaming, lack of motivation, impaired judgment, being unable to concentrate
- *Physical/sensations* – Numbness, headache, tiredness, nausea, loss of appetite, insomnia, muscular tension, pain, shortness of breath
- *Behavioral/actions* – Crying, social withdrawal, changes in activity level, avoidance of places or reminders, sleep disturbances, restless overactivity
- *Spiritual/existential* – Deepening of faith as source of strength, questioning/rethinking basic beliefs about faith, anger at G/god(s), confronting existential questions (Who am I? Why am I here? Where am I going?)

Making Time and Space for Loss and Grief in Sessions

Information predominates the era of genomics, and it can seem that there is no time to attend to loss and grief. Based on repeated client report that the human aspects of care are most important, time and space need to be made. Practitioners are encouraged to explore and potentially lower their level of verbal dominance in sessions and reduce the amount of information being provided in order to create space. Quite a bit can be accomplished in under 10 minutes.

There can also be hesitation about potentially upsetting clients by raising these top-ics. When explored, this concern is often rooted in the counselor's desire to be liked by clients, fear of employing empathic challenge, and/or the counselor being uncomfortable with loss and grief. In these cases, practitioners may be responding to their own needs rather than the client's. In addition to exploring the strategies provided in this chapter, it can be helpful to recall that if you raise something the client is not open to, they will let you know, and you can move on without disruption to the relationship.

Learning the Map

Two of the most comprehensive and influential grief theories currently are Stroebe and Schut's Dual-Process Model shown in Figure 5.1 and Worden's Tasks of Mourning shown in Figure 5.2, both of which can be used to enhance client self-efficacy and guide counselor interventions. Coupled with theories about

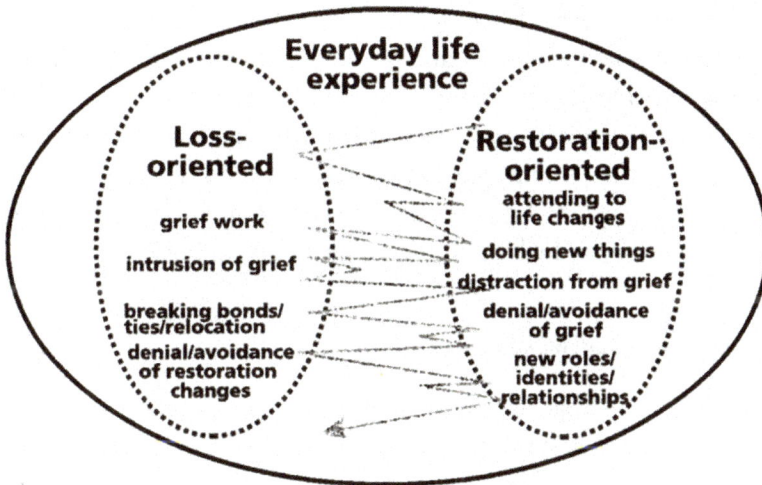

Figure 5.1   Stroebe and Schut's Dual Process Model (From Stroebe and Schut 1999, with permission.)

Figure 5.2   Worden's Tasks of Mourning

adaptation, coping, and Rolland's Family Systems Illness Model, genetic counselors can have a strong understanding of the framework of loss and grief to support their work with clients. Practitioners unfamiliar with more recent grief models and other theories mentioned may benefit from reviewing the ample publications available on these topics.

As you are more familiar with the landscape of loss and grief, you can bring more intentionality to your interventions with skills that you already have. Simple interventions, when offered with compassion in a supportive space, can be very powerful:

- *Listen:* Elicit client narratives and actively listen for loss and grief
- *Make space:* Ask about the client's experience of loss and grief
- *Name:* Primary and key secondary losses
- *Validate:* Normalize the client's experience of loss and grief
- *Recognize and reflect back:* Meaning reconstruction is a critical aspect of adaptation for most grieving people, and providing positive reinforcement of these efforts can be helpful
- *Identify sources of support:* Ask clients what/who they are finding valuable in their grief; help them invite more of these into their life
- *Identify gaps in support:* Ask clients what/who is missing in their grief, help them consider how and where they could get this support

Intercultural Communication around Loss and Grief

We all belong to groups that have norms about how to grieve. It is important to be aware of our own cultural assumptions about grief in order to recognize that they may not be shared by our clients. Counselors can engage self-reflection and self-education tools about norms related to grief and culture to raise their level of awareness about their own assumptions. When engaging clients in intercultural communication about loss and grief, consider exploring some of the following to further tailor your interventions and support:

- What is most valued, autonomy or connectedness?
- Who/What should be grieved?
- What obligations are felt to fulfill community responsibilities? To work through grief?
- Should emotions be expressed or contained? And where and when should they be expressed or contained?
- Do religion or other dominant belief systems normalize or pathologize loss and suffering? Does the client's story find a place within their dominant cultural narratives? Does their religion support, oppress, or marginalize their grief?

Knowing When to Refer

Genetic counselors provide short-term, client-centered counseling. Clients desiring support in their loss and grief beyond the time frame of genetic counseling can be referred for continuing care.

It can be helpful to identify if a client's grief lasts longer than expected based on social, cultural, or religious norms. For most clients, symptoms of grief begin to decrease over time following a loss, but for a small group, intense grief can remain and continue to negatively affect everyday functioning. Prolonged grief disorder was added to the *Diagnostic and Statistical Manual of Mental Disorders*, Fifth Edition in 2021. It is characterized by recurrent feelings including:

- *Identity disruption* (such as feeling as though part of oneself has died)
- *Intense emotional pain* (such as anger, bitterness, sorrow) related to a loss
- *Difficulty with reintegration* (such as problems engaging with friends, pursuing interests, planning for the future)
- *Emotional numbness* (absence or marked reduction of emotional experience)
- *Feeling that life is meaningless*
- *Intense loneliness* (feeling alone or detached from others)

Approximately 7% to 10% of people may experience symptoms of prolonged grief disorder following a significant loss, such as death of a loved one. This number can be higher in certain populations – one study found that 42% of people who witnessed the death of a person with an inherited cardiovascular disease experienced prolonged grief. Prolonged grief requires the intervention of a clinical psychologist or psychiatrist. It can adversely affect health outcomes, increasing the risk for suicide and psychological conditions such as depression and posttraumatic stress disorder. Individuals at higher risk of developing prolonged grief include older adults, caregivers of someone who died, people with a history of depression or bipolar disorder, and when the death of a loved one happens suddenly or under traumatic circumstances.

As genetic counselors in the era of genomics, we have a responsibility to develop our comfort with loss and grief, our understanding of these experiences, and our skills to provide support and facilitation for our clients. This work distinguishes us among genetic service providers and requires continued personal and professional growth throughout our careers.

Case Study

Amir sees Camila, a 16 year old with epilepsy, who is referred by her neurologist for genetic testing. During case prep, Amir notes Camila's developmental stage of adolescence and recalls that she is likely motivated toward greater independence from her family and a wider social network. He sees that Camila has been trialed on a variety of anti-epileptic medications but continues to have occasional breakthrough seizures. Amir wonders if, because of her intractable epilepsy, Camila has experienced any loss of independence or experiences she was anticipating for this time of her life. Amir decides to reserve a few minutes to explore these topics with Camila and her family. He also notes from the chart that Camila has self-identified as Catholic and that she immigrated from Colombia with her family when she was 2. Amir recognizes these are aspects of identity that he does not share and that could impact her experience of loss and grief. He takes a few minutes to identify how his culture and belief systems inform his views on loss and grief so he can avoid his assumptions overtly influencing the session.

Initially, Camila is talkative as Amir builds rapport by asking about her favorite subjects in school and the band T-shirt she is wearing as well as when he takes a family history. Following the medical history, Amir asks how she has been coping with all of the appointments, medications, and breakthrough seizures. Camila becomes quiet and appears somewhat sad. Amir notices the clock on the wall and quickly reviews his agenda in his head – he still has to introduce and explain exome sequencing, review possible results and impacts on management, explore the family's interest in pursuing testing, and potentially obtain consent and collect samples. He recognizes that prioritizing a working relationship with Camila is central to everything else he will undertake with this family and chooses to engage loss and grief before moving ahead.

Amir reflects to Camila that she has become quieter and seems sad, and he wonders out loud if this has to do with talking about how epilepsy is impacting her life recently. She nods slowly yes and glances to her parents. Amir addresses Camila and her parents by explaining that the emotional journey is just as important in genetic counseling as the medical journey. Her parents appear relieved and share how hard the past year has been for them as they have tried their best to support her. Camila then shares that what she really wants is to have a sleepover with her friends after the dance at school coming up, but her parents worry about her safety, and she also doesn't want to have a seizure in front of her friends.

Amir names Camila's loss of independence at a time in life when it is particularly important for her to be developing relationships with friends. He also names the loss of control and the feelings of helplessness her parents describe. He goes on to validate all of this as a very difficult but normal part of being this age and learning to live with epilepsy. He also names the love that they seem to have for each other and the strong bonds within their family. They all agree. Amir then identifies for the family that they seem to be on a journey that may not have a near-term end, even if they pursue genetic testing. He asks what has been most helpful to them each during this time and reflects back the strength and courage they are demonstrating. Amir then suggests that after the session, they consider how they might accommodate the upcoming sleepover to balance Camila's emerging independence and her safety as a start to the many other decisions they will make together as she becomes a young adult. They agree. Amir prepares to transition into talking about testing options and glances at the clock again. It has been 8 minutes.

Later that evening, Amir reflects on the case and considers the differences in how he and his family would have navigated a similar circumstance. He offers silent gratitude for his parents and his health and also hope for Camila and her family. He makes a note on his work calendar to check in with them in 2 weeks to see how their conversations went. He explores his own feelings and notices a bit of uncertainty about working with adolescents, which is less familiar to him. He decides to review the case with his colleagues this week as an opening for them to consider how their clinic might best support transition to adulthood with a chronic medical condition.

KEY POINT SUMMARY

- Loss and grief are central to our work with genetic counseling clients.
- Understanding of human loss and grief has evolved significantly in recent decades.
- While loss is a shared human experience, the experience of loss and grief is unique for each client.
- Loss and grief have the potential to create growth for clients. Our role is to facilitate this.
- Our own discomfort with loss and grief can limit our capacity to support clients and train students.
- Making time and space in sessions for loss and grief does not take long.
- Simple interventions using skills we already have can be powerful.
- Become aware of your cultural assumptions about grief and recognize that they may not be shared by clients.
- Referral for ongoing grief support as well as possible prolonged grief may be appropriate.

Bibliography

Ashtiani S et al. Parents' experiences of receiving their child's genetic diagnosis: A qualitative study to inform clinical genetics practice. *Am J Med Genet A*. 2014;164A:1496–1502.

Bernhardt BA et al. Distress and burnout among genetic service clinicians. *Genet Med*. 2009;11:527–535.

Douglas HA. Promoting meaning-making to help our patients grieve: An exemplar for genetic counselors and other health care professionals. *J Genet Couns*. 2014;23(5):695–700.

Edwards A et al. Interventions to improve risk communication in clinical genetics: Systematic review. *Patient Educ Couns*. 2008;71:4–25.

Fujisawa D et al. Prevalence and determinants of complicated grief in general population. *J Affect Disord*. 2010;127:352–358.

Geller G et al. Genetics professionals' experiences with grief and loss: Implications for support and training. *Clin Genet*. 2010;77(5):421–429.

Humphrey KM. *Counseling Strategies for Loss and Grief.* American Counseling Association, 2009.

Ingles J et al. Posttraumatic stress and prolonged grief after the sudden cardiac death of a young relative. *JAMA Intern Med*. 2016;176:402–405.

Kessler S. Psychological aspects of genetic counseling, IX. Teaching and counseling. *J Genet Couns*. 1997;6(3):287–295.

Klass D et al., eds. *Continuing Bonds: New Understandings of Grief*. Taylor & Francis, 1996.

Kübler-Ross E. *On Death and Dying*. Scribner, 1969.

Levine S. *Meetings at the Edge: Dialogues with the Grieving and the Dying, the Healing and the Healed*. Gateway, 1984.

Macnamara EF et al. Cases from the Undiagnosed Diseases Network: The continued value of counseling skills in a new genomic era. *J Genet Couns*. 2019;28(2):194–201.

Neimeyer RA et al. Grief therapy and the reconstruction of meaning: From principles to practice. *J Contemp Psychother*. 2010;40:73–83.

Prigerson HG et al. Traumatic grief as a risk factor for mental and physical morbidity. *Am J Psychiatry*. 1997;154:616–623.

Rolland JS. *Helping Couples and Families Navigate Illness and Disability: An Integrated Approach*. Guilford Press, 2018.

Smith C et al. The impact of genetic counseling on women's grief and coping following termination of pregnancy for fetal anomaly. *J Genet Couns*. 2021;30(2):522–532.

Spencer A. Stories as gift: Patient narratives and the development of empathy. *J Genet Couns*. 2016;25(4):687–690.

Stroebe M, Schut H. The dual process model of coping with bereavement: Rationale and description. *Death Stud*. 1999;23(3):197–224.

Szuhany KL et al. Prolonged grief disorder: Course, diagnosis, assessment, and treatment. *Focus (Am Psychiatr Publ)*. 2021;19(2):161–172.

Walter T. Grief and culture: A checklist. *Bereavement Care*. 2010;29(2):5–9.

Worden JW. *Grief Counseling and Grief Therapy: A Handbook for the Mental Health Practitioner*. Springer, 2009.

6

COUNTERTRANSFERENCE

MICHELLE E. FLORIDO

Introduction

The term "countertransference" was first introduced by Sigmund Freud in the 1900s and today is considered a foundational element of psychotherapy. The notion of countertransference was originally introduced in relation to the phenomenon of transference, whereby clients respond to providers in a way that is driven by their history of relating to others. Transference involves unconscious assumptions and misunderstandings that can lead to strong and often misplaced reactions toward the provider. Whereas transference encompasses a client's response to a provider, countertransference is the provider's response to a client.

Genetic counselors may experience countertransference in response to a client's life circumstances, personality traits, physical appearance, and/or other characteristics and can be influenced by the counselor's own positionality and demeanor. There may be times when a genetic counselor can anticipate a potential countertransference reaction due to clear and obvious similarities between the counselor and client, such as a shared age, identity, or medical/family health history. Other times, countertransference can occur without warning and may originate from deep within the recesses of the counselor's psyche as a reflexive response to past experiences, feelings, or circumstances. In either situation, it is important for genetic counselors to develop a level of self-awareness in order to identify the signs of a countertransference response, even if it may not be immediately clear what is evoking the reaction. Of note, not all emotions and responses on the part of the counselor represent countertransference; it is important to identify what is countertransference and what represents a genuine response.

Types of Countertransference

Two main types of countertransference described by Kessler (1992) are associative and projective countertransference. Associative countertransference refers to situations in which the genetic counselor loses focus on the client and instead turns inward toward their own feelings and thoughts. For example, a prenatal genetic counselor who recently discovered they are pregnant may experience associative countertransference when meeting with a client whose NIPT was positive for trisomy 21; the counselor may find themselves carried into their own thoughts, wondering how they might

DOI: 10.1201/9781003397847-6

feel, respond to and navigate such information about their own pregnancy. Projective countertransference occurs when the genetic counselor makes an assumption about the client's experience. This may be based on how the counselor has felt (or believes they would feel) in a similar situation or how someone else has described feeling and is not based on evidence offered by the client. For example, a genetic counselor whose mother was diagnosed with ovarian cancer in the past may experience projective countertransference when meeting with a client whose mother was recently diagnosed with ovarian cancer; the genetic counselor may recall their own thoughts, feelings, and reactions to their mother's diagnosis and assume the experience of their client is the same without using their assessment skills to learn about this from the client directly. These assumptions create a missed opportunity for connection and understanding, and without assessing the client's emotions, fears, values, and priorities, they might inhibit the counselor from effectively facilitating decision-making that aligns with the client's goals; furthermore, it may preclude therapeutic support that is in alignment with the client's emotions, experiences, and needs.

As outlined by Watkins (1985), countertransference can also be benign, overprotective, rejecting, or hostile. Benign countertransference occurs when the genetic counselor limits exploration of difficult feelings and topics, generally in response to a strong need to be liked and fear of negative patient emotions. This may be more likely to occur in trainees and newer genetic counselors who are in the process of building confidence in their abilities to share difficult information or reflect difficult truths back to clients and therefore fawn in the face of being viewed as the 'bearer of bad news'. With overprotective countertransference, the counselor may soften difficult information and/or spend excess time worrying about a client. Countertransference can also be rejecting, in which the counselor engages in ways that create distance with the client, or hostile, in which case the counselor experiences dislike toward a client and responds in a way that is harsh (either overtly or subliminally). Reeder et al. (2017) studied types of countertransference responses common in genetic counselors and subsequently described three tendencies: control – in which the counselor dislikes uncertainty/ambiguity (and the associated client emotions) and thus seeks to maintain or regain control; conflict avoidance – whereby the counselor is uncomfortable with confrontation and strong affect and seeks to avoid both; and directiveness – where the counselor pushes the client to make a decision that aligns with their own values, time frame, and/or decision-making style.

While countertransference is universally inevitable, it can prevent the counselor from being able to provide counseling that is truly client centered if it is not readily identified and appropriately navigated; instead, it may shift focus away from the client to the counselor, allow for unconscious assumptions, and/or blur important professional boundaries. This all, in turn, can inhibit the counselor's ability to effectively see, understand, validate, and support the client. Understanding the types of countertransference and being able to recognize when it is occurring are important steps toward mitigating these challenges.

Challenges and Strategies

Recognizing Common Causes of Countertransference

There are a variety of circumstances that might lead to a countertransference response. One of the most common is meeting with a client who, in some way, feels familiar to the counselor – this might be through a physical resemblance, mannerism, shared identity, cadence of speech, common background, or other similarity. Countertransference might also occur when a client is in a similar life stage or shares a common identity with the counselor. Having multiple shared identities with a client, particularly if there are specific circumstances shared between the counselor and client, can be more likely to lead the counselor to overidentify with a client. Conversely, countertransference can also occur when a counselor perceives that they are very dissimilar from a client; with a perceived chasm between the genetic counselor and client, the genetic counselor may pull further away and disengage from the client rather than doing the work of assessing and understanding the client and their circumstances. Other causes of countertransference can occur in relation to a counselor's own family dynamics, particularly from their childhood; past lived experiences; significant life events (e.g., pregnancy); topics that are personally challenging (e.g., religion, death, domestic violence); and tasks that may be perceived as difficult (e.g., giving bad news, working with children and adolescents).

Identifying Signs of Countertransference

There are a variety of ways in which a genetic counselor might identify that they are experiencing countertransference. These include:

- Feeling especially anxious or excited about meeting with a client
- Being carried into one's inner thoughts during a client encounter
- Noticing an atypical physical response during an encounter (e.g., heart racing, stomach in knots)
- Assumed understanding of a client's lived experience without assessing what is true for the client
- Feeling the urge to share personal life details beyond what is typical
- Wanting to end the session as quickly as possible or to prolong the session
- Feeling compelled to ensure the counselor is liked and seen positively by the client
- Experiencing intense and/or prolonged emotions (e.g., despair, anger, sadness, grief, happiness, etc.) related to a client or their situation
- Feeling apathetic to, indifferent toward, and/or disinterested in a client
- Having a response to a client that is exaggerated in light of the circumstances
- Feeling compelled to go above and beyond for a client, in particular when going past established client–counselor boundaries
- Feeling overprotective and/or that the counselor is the only one able to help, fix, or 'save' the client

Impact of Countertransference – Consequences

While countertransference is commonly experienced by genetic counselors, it is not always recognized. When it goes unnoticed by the genetic counselor, there are potential consequences that might occur and can impact the working relationship with the client. The main consequences of unrecognized and unchecked countertransference include overidentification, blurred boundaries, and a shift away from client-centered counseling. For example, a genetic counselor experiencing countertransference might feel compelled to overshare personal anecdotes and potentially (and often unintentionally) shift focus away from the client and onto the self; this may occur to such a degree that the client feels compelled to comfort the counselor. In some circumstances, the counselor might unintentionally assume an understanding of the client's values, goals, priorities, decision-making process, expectations, hopes, and emotional response; by assuming rather than assessing, there is a lost opportunity to connect with the client and provide care that centers the client and their needs. In other situations, the counselor may avoid certain topics altogether that they perceive to be painful or anticipate would elicit difficult and/or strong emotions. Boundaries may also become blurred; the counselor might go out of their way to help a client beyond what is typical or within reason. This can be the result of overidentification with the client and emotional nearness to the situation, which clouds judgment and makes the counselor a less objective and ultimately less effective provider. Ultimately, chronic overidentification and enmeshment with clients can increase the likelihood that a genetic counselor will experience professional burnout. When countertransference is identified and navigated appropriately by the counselor, it can allow for heightened empathic attunement and personal growth.

Strategies   A universal truth about countertransference is that it cannot be avoided. While we do our best to separate the personal and professional and to establish healthy boundaries for our practice, we are nonetheless human and have decades of complex lived experiences, unconscious biases, and nuanced emotional responses informing the way we see and respond to others. There are a variety of ways that genetic counselors might navigate countertransference, many of which require a level of self-awareness and an ability to self-reflect and process. Such strategies include:

- Reflecting on past life experiences and relational dynamics, current life stage, and significant life events and considering how these might impact client dynamics
- Being in touch with the inner self and identifying what types of clients are likely to elicit a countertransference response at baseline
- Becoming familiar with the signs of countertransference and working on identifying these as they occur in real time
- Using cognitive strategies to remember the client is a unique individual with their own rich and complex history, refocusing on the client and their needs, and calling upon client-centered counseling skills

- Processing the emotional response to a particular client through journaling or other forms of written reflection
- Confiding in and debriefing with trusted colleagues
- Meeting with peers in a supervision group, with or without facilitation
- Establishing care with a therapist who can provide long-term support to unpack and process past life experiences

Case Study

Kendra was a 32-year-old cancer genetic counselor with 7 years of experience. She met with a 25-year-old client, Rose, who was referred due to a family history of a *BRCA1* pathogenic variant. Upon meeting for the first time, Kendra felt an immediate affinity toward Rose and found herself really wanting Rose to like her. When Rose expressed feeling fearful and anxious about the testing, Kendra downplayed the cancer risks and subsequent medical management in order to comfort Rose. She also surprised herself by giving Rose her personal phone number and offering for her to check in any time. Thereafter, she found herself wondering how Rose was doing and fantasizing that Rose had raved to her family and friends about what a great experience she had with Kendra and how kind and helpful she was.

As someone who normally had healthy boundaries with clients, Kendra was able to reflect that she was responding to and interacting with Rose differently. The interaction sat with her for days, and she could not pinpoint the source of this intense need to be liked by and care for Rose. She spent time reflecting on the encounter and examined what it was about Rose that made her feel this way. She hypothesized that perhaps it was their proximal life stage but thought it unlikely given that she often counseled women in their mid-20s and had never had this particular response.

Kendra was part of a peer supervision group and elected to share the details of the case with the other genetic counselors in her group. She invited questions to better understand the psychological underpinnings of her strong reactions. Throughout the course of an hour-long conversation, one of her peers offered that the way in which Kendra described her urge to protect and support Rose had parallels to a sibling relationship. Kendra initially dismissed this hypothesis because she was an only child. However, upon further discussion, it was elicited that Rose reminded Kendra of a young camper she had built a strong relationship with during her time as a counselor at a sleepaway camp; the camper had been anxious about being away from family, and Kendra had offered her comfort and taken on a "big sister" role. Through reflection and processing, Kendra was able to identify that Rose's looks and cadence of speech felt familiar and reminiscent of that young camper and evoked an unconscious reflexive response in Kendra. Upon identifying this, Kendra was able to appreciate that Rose and the camper were two distinct individuals and felt better equipped to realign her role as Rose's genetic counselor and to engage appropriately within that boundary.

KEY POINT SUMMARY

- Countertransference refers to a genetic counselor's response to a client that is rooted in the counselor's own past experiences and is a common, normal, and inevitable occurrence.
- When countertransference goes unrecognized, there is a potential for a negative impact on the therapeutic relationship that can manifest through overidentification, missed opportunities for connection, and/or blurred relational boundaries.
- Through attunement, self-reflection, and processing with appropriate personnel, genetic counselors can become skilled at recognizing and deftly navigating countertransference.

Bibliography

Abrams LK, Kessler S. The inner world of the genetic counselor. *J Genetic Couns*. 2002;22(1):5–17. https://doi:10.1023/A:1013864330624

Benoit LG et al. When you care enough to do your very best: Genetic counselor experiences of compassion fatigue. *J Genet Couns*. 2007;16(3):299–312. https://doi:10.1007/s10897-006-9072-1

Biesecker B. Genetic counseling and the central tenets of practice. *Cold Spring Harb Perspect Med*. 2020;10(3):a038968. https://doi:10.1101/cshperspect.a038968

Bosco AF. Caring for the care-giver: The benefit of a peer supervision group. *J Genet Couns*. 2000;9(5):425–430. https://doi.org/10.1023/A:1009458316485

Evans C. *Genetic Counseling: A Psychological Approach*. Cambridge University Press, 2006.

Hiller E, Rosenfield JM. The experience of leader-led peer supervision: Genetic counselors' perspectives. *J Genet Couns*. 2000;(9)5:399–410. https://doi:10.1023/A:1009402231506

Hyatt J. Countertransference in the genetic counseling setting: One counselor's personal journey. *J Genet Counsel*. 2012;21(2):197–198. https://doi:10.1007/s10897-011-9435-0

Kennedy AL. Supervision for practicing genetic counselors: An overview of models. *J Genet Couns*. 2000;9(5):379–390. https://doi:10.1023/A:1009498030597

Kessler S. Psychological aspects of genetic counseling. VIII. Suffering and countertransference. *J Genet Couns*. 1992;1(4):303–308. https://doi.org/10.1007/BF00962826

Likhite ML. The interface between countertransference and projective identification in a case presented to peer supervision. *J Genet Couns*. 2000;9(5):417–424. https://doi.org/10.1023/A:1009406332414

Matloff E. Becoming a daughter. *J Genet Counsel*. 2006;15(3):139–144. https://doi:10.1007/s10897-005-9012-5

McCarthy Veach P et al. *Facilitating the Genetic Counseling Process: Practice Based Skills*. 2nd edn. Springer, 2018.

Redlinger-Grosse K. Countertransference: Making the unconscious conscious. In: Leroy BS et al., eds., *Genetic Counseling Practice: Advanced Concepts and Skills*, 2nd edn. Wiley Blackwell, 2021.

Reeder R et al. Characterizing clinical genetic counselors' countertransference experiences: An exploratory study. *J Genetic Couns*. 2017;26(5):934–947. https://doi:10.1007/s10897-016-0063-6

Thomas BC et al. Is self-disclosure part of the genetic counselor's clinical role? *J Genetic Couns.* 2006;15(3):163–177. https://doi.org/10.1007/s10897-006-9022-y

Watkins CE. Countertransference: Its impact on the counseling situation. *J Couns Dev.* 1985;63(6): 356–359. https://doi.org/10.1002/j.1556-6676.1985.tb02718.x

Weil J. *Psychosocial Genetic Counseling.* Oxford University Press, 2000.

Weil J. Countertransference: Making the unconscious conscious. In: LeRoy BS et al., eds., *Genetic Counseling Practice: Advanced Concepts and Skills.* Wiley Blackwell, 2010.

7

Challenges to Student Training in the Genomic Era

ELANA LEVINSON

Introduction

The Genomic Era

The Human Genome Project's completion in 2003 marked the beginning of the genomic era, which has seen major breakthroughs in understanding genetic contributions to health and disease. Advances in technology now enable whole exome and genome sequencing, allowing for personalized medical care and treatment based on genetic profiles. Costs of genetic tests have decreased, making them more accessible, and genetic testing has become more routine, often being ordered by nongenetic providers. Direct-to-consumer genomics has also raised public awareness of and access to genetic testing, albeit often in the context of ancestry or "recreational genetics." Genetic counselors play a vital role in educating patients about genetic technologies and facilitating informed decision-making. However, this era presents challenges for genetic counseling training programs, which must increase diversity in the field, tailor teaching and feedback to meet the learning styles of their students, and provide cutting-edge didactic and fieldwork opportunities.

Students of the Genomic Era

Generations are shaped by historical and cultural influences, which impact their worldview. These characteristics inform how individuals interact with and experience the world around them. Before exploring the challenges that arise in teaching and supervising genetic counseling graduate students in the genomic era, we first need to understand more about these students and the world in which they live. Most current genetic counseling students are Millennials or Generation Z. Millennials (born 1981–1996) are tech savvy, globally connected, and value immediacy, authenticity, and trust. They grew up with computers in schools and are effective at both online and in-person communication. Generation Z (also called Gen Z; born 1997–2012) is the most racially and ethnically diverse generation. They are true digital natives in that they are the first to have grown up with access to the internet, digital technology, and smartphones. While they excel at multitasking, they have short attention spans and

 DOI: 10.1201/9781003397847-7

struggle with face-to-face communication. Given the global communities that they engage with, both Millennials and Gen Z tend to be more welcoming towards diversity and engage in social activism. They seek truth, are not afraid to identify social injustices, and advocate for equity.

In contrast, senior educators are Baby Boomers (born 1946–1964) or Generation X (born 1965–1980). These individuals were educated in an age when classes were taught entirely in person, studying was done from textbooks, and resources were gathered by physically going to the library. While educators are adapting to the digital age, it is not how they experienced education.

Challenges and Strategies

Bridging the Generational Gap in Learning and Teaching

There are inherent generational gaps in learning, teaching, and feedback practices. Today's educators are challenged to keep students interested and engaged in course content and classroom learning. They are concerned about student recall and retention of material and notice a decline in mastery of skills. Educators need to better understand today's digital learners and adapt teaching styles to connect with them more effectively.

Millennial and Gen Z students are effective visual learners and prefer a blended learning approach, prioritizing active and visual learning, over passive learning. With this in mind, educators can consider turning traditional lectures into dynamic activities. Lecture materials should be visually attractive, using presentation software and incorporating images and graphs. Active listening can be encouraged by teaching in short bursts and weaving in case-based stories and interactive activities, supporting student desires for participatory, collaborative tasks that involve real-world applications. Learning materials can include a mix of digital reading, podcasts, and short videos. Students can also be encouraged to stay engaged in and outside the classroom with use of interactive polling systems and online discussion boards. Taking it one step further, a flipped-classroom approach delivers didactic content asynchronously, allowing students to digest content at their own pace, and uses classroom time for discussion and application of that content. In clinical fieldwork training, students appreciate opportunities to practice counseling in simulated sessions, which can be recorded, reviewed, and reflected upon to enhance learning.

Millennial and Gen Z students want clear expectations and feedback that is constructive, open, and immediate. Course instructors should review syllabi to ensure that expectations are stated in writing, and these should be discussed at the beginning and/or throughout the course. Students and instructors may also appreciate the opportunity to co-create community agreements, creating space for both students and instructors to voice expectations and needs. Instructors should provide clear criteria for how learning is assessed and strive to provide feedback in a timely manner. In some instances, it may be helpful to provide assessment rubrics for maximum transparency. Fieldwork supervisors should provide appreciative and constructive feedback after each counseling session or at the end of each day rather than after longer stretches of time. Direct observation tools, called workplace-based assessments (WBAs), may be helpful in providing quick formative feedback to students and used to prompt and guide further discussion of skills and competencies.

Keeping Pace with Genetic and Genomic Technologies

Advances in technology and science push the boundaries and change the landscape of genomic services. Genetic counselors need to be well equipped and knowledgeable about new technologies and their application to patient care. A recent study shows many genetic counselors feel they lack the training on genomic technologies that they need to perform their jobs. Genetic counseling programs are challenged to stay abreast.

The 2023 Standards of Accreditation for graduate programs in genetic counseling, as published by the Accreditation Council for Genetic Counseling (ACGC), require that graduate education include training on personalized genomic medicine, variant classification, and interpretation as well as use of bioinformatics and computerized tools. To provide this training, graduate programs need faculty with expertise in these areas to develop courses and teach their students. With resources often at a minimum, there are several creative ways to address these challenges. Curriculum sharing offers one potential strategy, by which programs can share teaching resources. This practice already exists informally, where programs may pool resources like syllabi, evaluation rubrics, or slide decks. This has been describe as beneficial because it fosters collaboration between programs and improves efficiency. Programs have also noted the downsides to resource sharing in that it detracts from the uniqueness of the contents as well as its authorship and ownership. A more formalized practice of resource sharing, where programs collaborate in creating and sharing course materials, can ease the burden and reduce the strain on individual programs to develop courses on similar topics.

Another approach is for an independent entity (e.g., National Society of Genetic Counselors [NSGC]) to identify subject matter experts to create educational content. In 2017, the NSGC Pharmacogenetics Working Group developed a standardized education module on pharmacogenetics. This was a flipped-classroom module in which learners worked through self-guided online content and then participated in interactive workshops. This leveraged the expertise of one group and provided accessible, standardized education across multiple programs.

Increasing Access to Training Opportunities

As genomic medicine advances, new specialties emerge within the field of genetic counseling. More genetic counselors are needed to meet patient demand and train students. When once the majority of genetic counselors practiced in patient-facing roles in reproductive, cancer, and pediatric genetics, genetic counselors now practice in a diverse and growing array of specialties, including cardiology, neurology, ophthalmology, nephrology, metabolic disease, consumer genomics, laboratory sciences, and research. Students desire exposure to these specialties. However, opportunities to train in emerging areas are often limited. In the past students who identified a unique experience in another part of the country had to coordinate a summer internship, potentially incurring additional travel and housing expenses. Now, and especially since the COVID pandemic, the widespread use of telemedicine makes it easier for students to gain training via remote, telemedicine internships. These internships can occur at any time of the year, allowing students to stay on campus and providing access to a greater number of students.

Creating even greater access to graduate education and fieldwork training, several universities now offer hybrid or online graduate training in genetic counseling. This allows for students to live wherever they like, potentially reducing housing costs and the overall cost of a graduate education. Graduate cohorts can be larger given that program size is not as reliant on ability to provide local fieldwork opportunities. With an online, remote model, programs can build their network of faculty and fieldwork supervisors from around the country or the world. This model may also meet Gen Z preferences for individualized and self-paced learning.

Promoting Diversity, Equity, Inclusion, and Justice (DEIJ)

Healthcare provider–patient congruency improves patient satisfaction and, in the field of genetic counseling, can improve access to and uptake of genetic services. It is widely acknowledged, however, that the genetic counseling workforce lacks the ethnic and racial diversity of the communities we serve. While attempts to increase diversity have been a priority since the 1990s, more needs to be done. Today's generation of learners, being more attuned to DEIJ principles, should help accelerate progress.

Strategies to increase diversity start with recruitment and increasing awareness of the profession among school-aged children. Genetic counselors and graduate programs should consider participating in career fairs in middle schools and high schools, especially in regions with underrepresented communities. Graduate programs should evaluate their admissions requirements such as GRE and GPA cutoffs and application fees and consider that these may unjustly favor certain applicants. Admissions committee members should be trained to recognize implicit biases that may affect how they review applications or interviewees. Promoting and modeling DEIJ is also of upmost importance in the classroom and throughout graduate training. Course directors should ensure a diversity of contributors in course materials and allocate class time to discuss topics surrounding equity. Faculty should also gain comfort in acknowledging when material is not inclusive, identifying and addressing health disparities. Fieldwork supervisors should model use of inclusive language and create equitable clinic resources. More research is needed to understand how discussions of personal identity impact mentoring and supervisory relationships.

Students, faculty, and program leadership are encouraged to have candid conversations and practice self-reflection about identities and positionality and how these influence our experiences and worldviews. Discussions should take place in safe, supportive, and respectful environments, acknowledging that we are all learners in this space and working together to promote and improve health equity.

Training the Genetic Counseling Graduate Program Network

Tackling the challenges and enabling the strategies presented in this chapter require thought, creativity, effort, and a dedicated network of program directors, course directors, supervisors, and mentors, all working toward common goals. Graduate program faculty need access to and protected time to learn pedagogical theories, teaching, and feedback practices to best support the students and meet these goals. The field of genetic counseling is an evolving discipline that requires career-long learning not only to master the current state of genomics but also to develop ways to connect with and train the next generation of students as they step forth into the workforce.

Case Study

The Midwest Genetic Counseling Graduate Program is a (fictional) program in America's Heartland. They rely on their small local network of genetic counselors to provide didactic training and clinical supervision. They feel pressure from university administration and the profession to grow their program, but size is limited by the dearth of genetic counseling services in the vicinity for clinical rotations. Their students also desire more training in variant interpretation, but the faculty bandwidth is stretched, and no one feels equipped to take this on. The program director contacts other programs to understand how they are navigating these issues, and an alliance forms. The Midwest Genetic Counseling Graduate Program is able to enroll their students in an online course on variant interpretation offered by another graduate program. They also identify laboratory genetic counselors with expertise in variant interpretation who create a remote internship experience for their students, where they are able to apply their learnings to real-world scenarios and gain exposure to industry jobs. Leveraging technology, online learning, and remote training allowed the Midwest Genetic Counseling Graduate Program to provide robust didactic and experiential training in variant interpretation. Building their network of internship opportunities also made it possible for them to admit more students in subsequent years. This creative and collaborative approach helped satisfy the needs of their students, the administration, and the profession.

KEY POINT SUMMARY

- Millennials and Gen Z prefer a blended learning approach with active and visual learning and opportunities for interactive, collaborative tasks.
- Resource sharing, use of standardized education modules, or massive online courses can enable training in emerging technologies and variant interpretation.
- Creative use of telemedicine and remote learning can increase access to genetic counseling education and fieldwork training.
- Efforts to increase diversity in genetic counseling as well as promote health equity for patients should be multipronged and be woven throughout recruitment, admissions, and training. These efforts have the downstream effects of improving access to and satisfaction with genetic services.

Bibliography

Abdul Kadir S. The use of social media in millennials' teaching and learning activities in design related course. *Environ-Behav Proc J*. 2020;5(13).

Bao AK et al. Reflections on diversity, equity, and inclusion in genetic counseling education. *J Genet Couns*. 2020;29(2):315–323.

Farwell Hagman KD et al. Facing the challenge of genetic counselors' need for rapid continuing education about genomic technologies. *J Genet Couns*. 2020;29(5):838–848.

Ingram Nissen T et al. Microlearning: Evidence-based education that is effective for busy professionals and short attention spans. *J Genet Couns*. 2023;00:1–6.

Macfadyen LP et al. A novel online genomic counseling and variant interpretation certificate: Learning design, learning analytics, and evaluation. *J Genet Couns*. 2023;00:1–8.

Marra M et al. Fellowships for genetic counselors: An emerging opportunity for additional training and specialization. *J Genet Couns*. 2023;32:1276–1279.

McEwen A, Jacobs C. Preparing the genetic counseling workforce for the future in Australasia. *J Genet Couns*. 2021;30(1):55–60.

Mercado J et al. A call for unity in DEIJ efforts using a proposed framework for education, recruitment, retainment, research, and active outreach (ERA) for genetic counselors in the United States. *J Genet Couns*. 2022;31(3):590–597.

Mohzan MAM, Zubir HA. Teaching the millennials: Implications on today's classrooms. *Universal J Educ Res*. 2019;7(9A):186–191.

Murphy EE et al. Genetic counseling graduate program faculty perspectives on sharing education materials among programs. *J Genet Couns*. 2023;00:1–10.

National Society of Genetic Counselors. *2023 Professional Status Survey [Internet]*. www.nsgc.org/Policy-Research-and-Publications/Professional-Status-Survey

Patch C, Middleton A. Genetic counselling in the era of genomic medicine. *Br Med Bull*. 2018;126(1):27–36.

Peplow K et al. Discussions of personal identity in genetic counseling supervision. *J Genet Couns*. 2023;00:1–12.

Shorey S et al. Learning styles, preferences and needs of Generation Z healthcare students: Scoping review. *Nurse Educ Pract*. 2021;57:1–11.

Szymkowiak A et al. Information technology and Gen Z: The role of teachers, the internet, and technology in the education of young people. *Technol Soc*. 2021;65:1–10.

Young JQ et al. Advancing workplace-based assessment in psychiatric education: Key design and implementation issues. *Psychiatr Clin North Am*. 2021;44(2):317–332.

COMMUNICATION AND DOCUMENTATION IN THE ELECTRONIC HEALTH RECORD

SARA M. BERGER

Introduction

The electronic health record (EHR) has transformed healthcare by supporting documentation, billing, and clinical care. First developed in the 1970s, EHR systems saw low adoption rates until the 2009 American Recovery and Reinvestment Act, which included the Health Information Technologies for Economic and Clinical Health (HITECH) Act as well as other public policies that encouraged the adoption and meaningful use of the EHR. National adoption rates have since increased to over 90%, but many institutions face challenges in maintaining and updating their EHR systems including costs, regulatory changes, and staff cooperation. A few vendors dominate the market for EHR systems, and it remains a considerable challenge, from both a financial and technological perspective, to keep up with emerging fields including telemedicine, artificial intelligence, and genomics.

The American College of Medical Genetics (ACMG) has a points-to-consider statement discussing the definition of the scope of genomic data within the EHR, the right of access to genomic data for the individual, genetic exceptionalism, and social justice concerns. It aims to assist clinicians, laboratories, institutions, and EHR vendors as they develop policies and procedures to optimize genomic data use within the EHR. Similarly, the Association for Molecular Pathology (AMP) offers perspectives relating to interoperability, challenges, opportunities, and solutions to address issues related to how genomic data is displayed and used within the EHR. They outline the workflow and data transformations required for the EHR to seamlessly integrate genomic data, interfacing with the laboratory information system, reference databases, clinical decision support tools, coverage/reimbursement databases, and both structured and unstructured patient data. The challenges and complexities that need to be addressed to be truly "genomics ready" are considerable.

This chapter discusses issues that clinicians may encounter in their use of the EHR as it relates to genetics and genomics.

DOI: 10.1201/9781003397847-8

Challenges and Strategies

Technical Challenges

There is significant potential in the integration and utilization of genomic data within the EHR but its usefulness for clinical decision-making and research is only as good as the data itself. Currently, most clinicians receive genetic test results from the laboratory as a PDF that is manually scanned into the EHR. In some cases, the laboratory can push the results directly to the EHR as a PDF or a flat text file. While PDF reports are ideal for patient-facing documentation, the data contained cannot be queried within the EHR. For the EHR to utilize the information contained in a genetic test report, the results must be received as discrete, individually coded data elements, which requires both the reporting laboratories and the EHR systems to adopt compatible data storage and exchange practices. Health Level 7 (HL7) Fast Healthcare Interoperability Resources (FHIR) standards are created by an accredited organization responsible for multiple information exchange standards, facilitating different systems to exchange information and agree on the meaning of each piece of data. The need to improve interoperability has been noted by both ACMG and AMP points to consider.

There are significant efforts in the field to address this challenge. The eMERGE Network phase III study aims to integrate genomic test results into the EHR by using HL7 FHIR standards. Their work contributed to the Genomics Reporting Implementation Guide, ensuring structured genomic result return with meaningful data elements while prioritizing the patient experience and not overburdening genetic testing laboratories.

However, technical challenges to interoperability remain the primary barrier to the utilization of genomic data within the EHR. Most institutions do not receive genomic data in a discrete form and are unable to use that data to query specific genes or variants. EHR systems were not designed for genomic data, making customization a technological and financial burden. Storage of genomic data adds further complexity, and most EHR systems operate with a main "package" that has optional add-on items which institutions pay for. Furthermore, variability in system capabilities can be seen across institutions with the same EHR due to differences in financial investment and governance policies.

Clinical Care

There is tremendous potential for the EHR to improve clinical care; however, there are many well-documented challenges and limitations. A 2021 study from the University of Pennsylvania grouped these into five main categories:

- *Usability and usefulness* – How easy is the EHR for the clinician to use?
- *Data quality* – How good is the data in the EHR?

- *Standards* – How does the EHR adhere to and reflect established standards?
- *Governance* – What policies are in place to ensure the EHR is used appropriately?
- *Data integration* – How is the data within the EHR connecting and communicating with other sources of data?

Each of these components intersects and impacts the use of the EHR, becoming increasingly complex when considering genomic data. For example, the EHR can be used to identify patients with a specific diagnosis and alert their healthcare providers to gaps in their care based on clinical guidelines. A data point is needed for the EHR to identify the diagnosis to trigger an alert to their provider. This could be from the problem list, a diagnosis code, a lab value, or another data point. However, many genetic conditions do not have a specific diagnosis code and often do not appear on the problem list.

One of the main advantages of the EHR is the ability to access a patient's records from other institutions, which improves consistency of clinical care and reduces redundant orders and procedures. However, inconsistencies in genetic testing ordering and storage (often as PDFs) complicates locating prior results, leading to unnecessary testing. While the EHR can pull lab values directly into documentation using a typed shortcut to reduce errors, including genomic data often requires retyping or copying from PDF reports, which is time-consuming and error-prone. It is important to always reference the original genetic test report and not to rely on the documentation of other clinicians about the gene, variant, or classification because this can amplify misinformation.

The complexity of genetic testing, including varied types of required samples, different technologies, and turnaround times, can compound challenges to manage and coordinate genetic testing for a single patient and may require duplicate efforts, in part due to the lack of integration of genetic testing orders and results within the EHR. Multiple groups are working on strategies to manage the genetics care coordination within their division or institution. Efforts like the University of Michigan's Pediatric Genetic Tracking module centralize a summary of the patient's genetic testing, follow-up, and diagnosis. This is visible to clinicians across the institution so they can see all the genetics care for a patient in one place instead of searching throughout the EHR. Similarly, the University of Pennsylvania demonstrated that linking genetic test orders and results to discrete data within the EHR resulted in a significant reduction in the time it takes to order a genetic test and manage the genetic test result.

The technological lift to integrate genetic and genomic information as discrete data across all laboratories and institutions is a heavy one with an indiscernible timeline. To ensure genetic testing and genomic data are the most impactful, it is important to order and store genetic and genomic data in a consistent way within an institution. Clinicians from different clinical areas who order genetic testing must collaborate with the laboratories, IT, and teams who collect, process, or send out the samples and results. Together, they should develop a system that is transparent and consistent so that every provider will know how to locate genetic testing that may have been done for a patient.

Family Member Records within the EHR

Genetic testing has significant impact not only on the patient who had the testing done but also on their family members. Genetic testing done for family members may be used in the care of a patient, but it can be a challenge to maintain the privacy and confidentiality of the family member's information when that information is added to the patient's EHR. Some EHR systems have the ability to link family member records, but it is not always clear to the patient or their clinician what information may be shared as a result of linking their charts.

Examples:

- A patient with a family history of breast cancer brings her oncologist a copy of her sister's genetic testing report with a pathogenic variant in *BRCA1*.
- A newborn baby is in the neonatal intensive care unit, and an amniocentesis done prenatally confirmed a diagnosis of trisomy 21; these records are in the mother's chart.
- A pregnant patient is found to be a carrier for spinal muscular atrophy, and her partner's carrier screening is negative.
- A patient with hearing loss has a variant of uncertain significance identified on a panel, and parental testing is done to confirm inheritance and aid in interpretation.
- Exome sequencing done for a patient with autism reports a paternally inherited secondary finding in the *MHY7* gene.

The inclusion or exclusion of the family member records from the patient's chart could have a significant impact on their clinical care. Lack of access to the family member's records can lead to incorrect or unnecessary genetic testing for a patient. However, protecting the privacy and confidentiality of the family member, especially when their records are identifiable (e.g., a genetic testing report with their name and date of birth), remains an important consideration. Additional privacy protection mechanisms could be used for these types of records, such as marking them as a separate document category that is secure or confidential or even limiting access to only specific clinicians. When doing follow-up testing for a partner, parent, or other family member based on the results of the patient, a chart for that family member should be created, and all records relevant to their testing should be documented in their own chart, even if it is being done to help interpret the significance of genetic testing results of the patient.

Ethical/Legal

While a primary goal of the EHR is to increase accessibility for patients and clinicians, there are still limitations. EHR systems generally operate in English, and while patient portal access may be available in multiple languages, the content of the records often remains in English. Accommodations for those who are visually or hearing impaired are limited. Using the EHR requires digital and data literacy as well as access. In order for the EHR to truly provide universal access to health data, including genomic data, we must consider issues related to access, literacy, knowledge, and awareness across communities.

The Office of the National Coordinator for Health Information Technology's 21st Century Cures Act includes the interoperability and information-blocking rules. This requires that patients and their representatives have immediate digital access to their electronic health information at no cost. Providers who are subject to this rule and do not share the information with the patient may be subject to penalties and disincentives. There are a limited number of exceptions, and based on this rule, many institutions' EHR automatically releases notes, laboratory results, and imaging reports unless they are subject to an exception. Therefore, it is possible that the patient or clinicians other than the ordering provider may see test results prior to the ordering provider contacting the patient to discuss the results. Some genetic test results pose more of a challenge in this space than others. It is important that this is discussed with the patient and their family when establishing a plan for results disclosure. It is also important to educate clinicians to refer to the notes from the ordering clinician regarding the results of the genetic testing and their interpretation instead of interpreting the significance of the genetic test results in a vacuum.

A common concern for patients regarding the EHR is privacy and who has access to their data. Patients have concerns about health insurance companies, pharmaceutical companies, government agencies, or other parties using their data and the risks of discrimination, stigmatization, or psychosocial distress if there is a breach of privacy. Patients and families should be aware of the nuances and challenges of genetic testing within the EHR, and institutions should develop transparent and consistent processes regarding display, access and storage of genetic information within the EHR.

KEY POINT SUMMARY

- Genomic data is often received as PDFs, making integration into the EHR challenging. Interoperability requires standardized formats like HL7 FHIR, but implementation is resource-intensive and varies across institutions.

- Inconsistent ordering and storage of genetic testing results lead to inefficiencies, redundant testing, and errors. Genomic data integration into clinical workflows remains labor-intensive and prone to inaccuracies.
- Incorporating family member genetic information into a patient's EHR poses risks to privacy and confidentiality, requiring careful handling and restricted access to sensitive data.
- Automatic release of genetic test results under regulations like the 21st Century Cures Act can result in patients or clinicians seeing sensitive results without adequate context, necessitating clear result disclosure planning.
- Barriers like language limitations, digital literacy, and access to EHRs disproportionately affect underserved populations, potentially widening healthcare disparities in the use of genomic data.

Bibliography

21st Century Cures Act. *Interoperability, Information Blocking, and the ONC Health IT Certification Program [Internet]*, 2020. www.federalregister.gov/documents/2020/05/01/2020–07419/21st-century-cures-act-interoperability-information-blocking-and-the-onc-health-it-certification

21st Century Cures Act. *Establishment of Disincentives for Health Care Providers That Have Committed Information Blocking [Internet]*, 2023. www.federalregister.gov/documents/2023/11/01/2023–24068/21st-century-cures-act-establishment-of-disincentives-for-health-care-providers-that-have-committed

Bombard Y et al. Digital health-enabled genomics: Opportunities and challenges. *Am J Hum Genet*. 2022;109(7):1190–1198.

Carter AB et al. Electronic health records and genomics: Perspectives from the Association for Molecular Pathology electronic health record (EHR) interoperability for clinical genomics data working group. *J Mol Diagnostics*. 2022;24(1):1–17.

Grebe TA et al. The interface of genomic information with the electronic health record: A points to consider statement of the American College of Medical Genetics and Genomics (ACMG). *Genet Med*. 2020;22(9):1431–1436.

Holmes JH et al. Why is the electronic health record so challenging for research and clinical care? *Methods Inf Med*. 2021;60(1–2):32–48.

Jiang J et al. Pre-pandemic assessment: A decade of progress in electronic health record adoption among U.S. hospitals. *Heal Aff Sch*. 2023;1(5):1–6.

Kanungo S et al. Ethical considerations on pediatric genetic testing results in electronic health records. *Appl Clin Inform*. 2020;11(5):755–763.

Lau-Min KS et al. From race-based to precision oncology: Leveraging behavioral economics and the electronic health record to advance health equity in cancer care. *JCO Precis Oncol*. 2021;(5):403–407.

Murugan M et al. Genomic considerations for FHIR®; eMERGE implementation lessons. *J Biomed Inform*. 2021;118:103795.

Raspa M et al. Preferences for accessing electronic health records for research purposes: Views of parents who have a child with a known or suspected genetic condition. *Value Heal*. 2020;23(12):1639–1652.

Scott A, Martin DM. Development and implementation of an electronic medical record module to track genetic testing results. *Genet Med*. 2021;23(5):972–975.

9

Obtaining Consent with Interpreters

NINA HARKAVY

Introduction

Genetic counseling requires clear communication of complex genomic concepts as well as emotional content, often more so than other types of medical encounters. There is a growing number of individuals in the United States with limited English proficiency (LEP), meaning a limited ability to speak, read, write, or understand English. The use of interpreters in healthcare settings is shown to improve health outcomes, patient knowledge, and patient satisfaction. Language interpretation in the setting of genetic counseling requires not only scientific vocabulary but also the ability to translate probabilistic statements and nuanced content. Previous studies have suggested that misinterpretations in genetic counseling negatively affect rapport building, patient understanding, and psychosocial assessment. These errors and limitations, in turn, affect our ability to obtain informed consent from patients. Browner et al. (2003), in their study of miscommunications in interpreted genetic counseling sessions, identified five common sources of miscommunication: medical jargon; the non-directive nature of counseling; the inhibitions of counselors stemming from misplaced cultural sensitivity; problems of translation; and problems of trust. Here, we discuss a number of challenges to obtaining informed consent with an interpreter and propose relevant strategies.

Challenges and Strategies

Ad Hoc versus Professional Interpreters

Interpreters in healthcare settings may be professionally trained or "ad hoc" untrained interpreters, often friends, family, or bilingual staff. A patient may state that they prefer their chosen ad hoc interpreter, and/or the provider may perceive it as easier than arranging a professional interpreter. However, the use of ad hoc interpreters has been associated with increased chances for miscommunication and reduced patient satisfaction, which may ultimately increase adverse outcomes. While some studies have found no significant difference in the *number* of errors between professional and ad hoc interpreters, there may be differences in the type and, most importantly, the

DOI: 10.1201/9781003397847-9

clinical significance of errors. It is also important to be aware of the regulations governing use of interpreters at one's workplace, as there may be recommendations or prohibitions against using untrained interpreters. Though it may seem that using an ad hoc interpreter is the more "efficient" choice, the increased chance for poor results and the amount of time that may be needed to clarify communications often negates any time or effort seemingly saved.

Miscommunication (Problems of Translation)

Flores et al. (2003) identified five categories of interpreter errors: omission, addition, substitution, editorialization, and false fluency. An omission error occurs when an interpreter does not interpret a word/phrase used by the speaker. An addition error occurs when an interpreter adds a word/phrase that was not used by the speaker. A substitution error is when a word/phrase is substituted for a different word/phrase not used by the speaker. Editorialization occurs when the interpreter provides their personal views instead of interpretation of the word/phrase used by the speaker. For example, if the patient asks a question that seems irrelevant to the interpreter, they say "your patient is confused." In false fluency, the interpreter uses an incorrect word/ phrase or uses a word/phrase that does not exist in the language. As an example of false fluency, if a Spanish interpreter refers to sickle cell disease as "*células sickle*," they are using a word, "sickle," that does not exist in Spanish rather than the medically accurate phrase "*células falciformes*."

A number of studies of Spanish interpretation in clinical settings have demonstrated the high frequency of errors even among trained interpreters. On average, studies have indicated 27 to 33 errors per clinical encounter. Errors can range in their clinical impact. While up to 77% of errors made by ad hoc interpreters have been reported to be clinically significant, more than 50% of the errors made by professional interpreters have also been found to be clinically significant. Omission errors are typically cited as the most frequent type of error.

There are a number of strategies that counselors can use to improve communication and reduce errors in their interpreted sessions. To promote faithful interpretation, use language that is clear and concise, remove filler words, and be direct with questions and observations. "Chunking," or providing small amounts of information with pauses rather than long explanations, helps to prevent errors of omission. Avoiding the use of colloquialisms or slang reduces false fluency errors (e.g., use "How are you feeling?" instead of "How is that sitting with you?"). While the use of some genetics jargon is unavoidable, all genetics terms should be clearly defined. The nongenetics vocabulary should also be modified for accessibility and ease of interpretation) (e.g., use "the chance for an extra chromosome is high" instead of "the probability for aneuploidy is elevated").

Confirming the patient's preferred language and specific dialect (e.g., Yemeni Arabic instead of Arabic) is a necessary step that can be overlooked. There are also nonverbal strategies to improve both communication and rapport, such as maintaining eye contact with the patient rather than with the interpreter or communication device. Finally, every statement in a session should be interpreted. If the interpreter and patient speak back and forth, the interpreter should provide an explanation of the exchange. Above all, counselors should remember that the role of the interpreter is to improve communication and ideally to serve as a cultural broker. *If a counselor is concerned about interpreter accuracy or appropriateness, it is both reasonable and ethical to request a new interpreter.* Counselors should feel empowered to ask interpreters clarifying questions about the content of an exchange and remind them to interpret all content. While counselors may worry about the added time to acquire a new interpreter or their own personal feelings of discomfort in requesting one, the harms of using an interpreter who is unclear, inaccurate, or impolite dramatically outweigh the benefits.

Culture and Power (Problems of Trust)

Problems of trust can exist in any counselor–patient interaction but may be exacerbated by an inability to communicate directly when language discordant. Ensuring accurate interpretation is important for the patient's perception of the session as much as for the counselor's. If a patient does not perceive that their words are being faithfully translated, they may feel disregarded. Similarly, asymmetric communication, in which a patient is implicitly asked to accept what the counselor says without being heard themselves, is also a source of miscommunication. In one recorded interaction from a study by Browner et al. (2003), a patient reflected after the session that she thought the counselor was not listening to her, saying, "Well, if she doesn't believe me, I don't believe her." Counselors may also experience hesitation to correct patients' mistaken beliefs for fear of cultural insensitivity and damaging rapport. However, rapport is only one of the means to the end of open communication; open communication should not be sacrificed to maintain rapport. Additionally, some patients may be used to a more "prescriptive" relationship with healthcare providers and are unfamiliar with the role of genetic counselors in supporting patient autonomy. Patients may interpret the "choice" to pursue intervention as necessarily meaning that the intervention is unimportant. Recognizing these potential cultural discrepancies, counselors should, at the beginning of the session, explain their role in helping patients navigate decisions. Genetic counselors may feel that they don't have time to prioritize two-way communication with a patient in interpreter-led sessions. Unsurprisingly, taking time to hear and check in with our patients only increases our ability to facilitate values-driven decision-making.

Effective Education

Ensuring informed consent requires that the provision of information by genetic counselors aligns with the informational needs of the patient. Working with interpreters necessitates that genetic counselors simplify their message while meeting the standards for informed consent. While many counselors would endorse the importance of explaining complex genetics concepts, the literature supports reducing the amount of information provided in order to highlight the most directly relevant information, especially as related to risk. Potential solutions include providing patients with informational resources in their primary language prior to an appointment to equip them with baseline information and/or provide postcounseling resources to reinforce genetics concepts. However, during the session, there is evidence for the value of focusing on the "minimum necessary" information. For example, in counseling a carrier–carrier couple, it may be more important to focus on 25% risk to offspring (and the couple's level of concern about the condition and risk) than to explain autosomal recessive inheritance in detail. Patients always have the option to request additional information if desired. Limiting the amount of new concepts taught in a session and identifying/reiterating the most significant "take-home" points improves patient understanding, especially in high-stress situations.

Patients with limited English proficiency may face additional cultural, language, or health literacy barriers compared to English-speaking patients. Trying to elicit understanding solely by asking the patient if they have any questions is flawed in that it does not address patients who are reluctant to ask, who don't know how to form their question, or who "don't know what they don't know." In addition to providing the "minimum necessary" information with an interpreter, the "teach-back" method supports health literacy and shared decision-making, both of which are essential components of informed consent. The teach-back method was created to improve provider–patient communication by allowing the provider to identify and correct misunderstood or incompletely understood information. The counselor frames the teach-back process to the patient to focus on the effectiveness of their own communication rather than the patient's ability to understand information (e.g., "I want to make sure I explained XYZ correctly"). The patient then verbalizes their understanding, allowing the counselor to clarify and potentially reteach concepts or to move forward in the consent process.

The onus of effective education does not rest exclusively on the individual genetic counselor or their patient. There is a lack of consistent standards for training, licensing, and certification of interpreters, which helps to explain the high rate of interpreter errors and variability in skill levels. While national regulations are difficult to directly address, clinics that frequently use interpreters for genetics consults can consider creating a tailored curriculum and/or providing bilingual genetics glossaries when possible (see, for example, Lexigene: https://www.lexigene.com/en/). Individual counselors can learn key terms and provide those to interpreters to correct mistakes in real time. Waggoner et al. (2023) demonstrated that genetic counselors with even basic Spanish proficiency can identify and correct a majority of clinically significant Spanish interpretation errors during a recorded session. The study concluded that language acquisition and familiarity, even without fluency, among genetic counselors improves our ability to offer equitable care to language-discordant patients. Support for language skill acquisition can be included as part of genetic counseling training curricula and/or continuing education for practicing counselors.

Case Study

A 30-year-old G1 pregnant patient and her partner are being seen for prenatal genetic counseling to review the patient's carrier status for cystic fibrosis (CF). The counselor explains that the patient is a carrier of CF and briefly describes CF as a serious genetic lung condition. The patient becomes tearful, explaining that she has asthma but is otherwise healthy. The counselor tries to reconcile the patient's affect and her sharing this information about her health. The counselor realizes that the interpreter may have stated that the patient "has" CF. She quickly clarifies that having the condition is not the same as being a carrier, emphasizing that carriers are typically asymptomatic. The patient expresses relief, and the counselor goes on to discuss carrier screening for the patient's partner. The couple agree that they would like to know the partner's carrier status so that they can make a decision about prenatal diagnosis. The counselor explains that the partner just has to sign a form, and then he can have his blood drawn. At this, the couple becomes quiet and looks nervously at one another. The partner shakes his head to indicate that he does not want to sign. The genetic counselor confirms again that the partner wants information about his own carrier status, then asks if something has made him uncomfortable. In their role as a cultural broker, the interpreter says to the counselor, "Excuse me, this is the interpreter speaking. I used the word 'paper' for 'form,' and I wonder whether your patient associates that term with immigration papers. Is it okay if I clarify with your patient that you are referring to a consent form?" The counselor agrees, and once interpreted, the partner agrees to sign and proceeds to the blood draw.

KEY POINT SUMMARY

- When possible, use professional rather than ad hoc interpreters to reduce the frequency of clinically significant errors.
- Provide information in small amounts ("chunks"), define all genetics vocabulary, and make an effort to use highly accessible language throughout the session. Avoid colloquialisms, slang, and nonliteral language.
- Speak directly to and maintain eye contact with patients. Prioritize two-way communication so that patients feel heard and thus more inclined to trust the counselor and the information provided.

- Plan to emphasize the "minimum necessary" information and key take-away points to reduce the amounts of new concepts that must be learned by a patient. Provide patients with educational resources in their language when possible.
- Switch interpreters if you sense that an interpreter is inaccurate or inappropriate; this reduces the risk for adverse outcomes.
- Practice "teach-backs" to ensure patient understanding and confirm informed consent.
- Advocate for genetics-specific language resources for interpreters (e.g., genetics glossaries) and provide language acquisition opportunities (e.g., language classes) for counselors and students to improve quality of care for non-English-speaking patients.

Bibliography

Browner CH et al. Genetic counseling gone awry: Miscommunication between prenatal genetic service providers and Mexican-origin clients. *Soc Sci Med.* 2003;56(9):1933–1946.

Cloutier M et al. Lexigene®: An online medical genetics translation tool to facilitate communication. *J Genet Couns.* 2019;28(3):717–721.

Flores G. The impact of medical interpreter services on the quality of health care: A systematic review. *Med Care Res Rev.* 2005;62(3):255–299.

Flores G et al. Errors in medical interpretation and their potential clinical consequences in pediatric encounters. *Pediatrics.* 2003;111(1):6.

Forrow L, Kontrimas JC. Language barriers, informed consent, and effective caregiving. *J Gen Intern Med.* 2017;32(8):855–857.

Gutierrez AM et al. Portero versus portador: Spanish interpretation of genomic terminology during whole exome sequencing results disclosure. *Pers Med.* 2017;14(6):503–514.

Joseph G, Guerra C. To worry or not to worry: Breast cancer genetic counseling communication with low-income Latina immigrants. *J Community Genet.* 2015;6(1):63–76.

Seely KD et al. Utilizing the "teach-back" method to improve surgical informed consent and shared decision-making: A review. *Patient Saf Surg.* 2022;16(1).

Waggoner RM et al. The utility of limited Spanish proficiency in interpreted genetic counseling sessions. *J Genet Couns.* 2023;32(3):663–673.

10

GENETIC TESTING FOR MINORS

MARGARET B. MENZEL

Introduction

Ethical issues surrounding genetic testing for minors has been an important focus of discussion and debate in healthcare since the 1950s, when karyotype analysis and then prenatal karyotyping (1960s) became available for children and fetuses. Genetic testing can benefit children in numerous ways, but it also has the potential to do harm. Appropriateness of testing, potential benefits and current or future harms, the consent process, and follow-up protocols are all important considerations in genetic testing of minors (Moore and Richer 2022). The genetic counselor plays a crucial role in the assessment of all of these as part of a multidisciplinary team. This chapter will review several key ethical considerations of genetic testing for minors and suggest strategies that genetic counselors may use to address them.

Assessing Whether Genetic Testing Is Appropriate for a Minor

Genetic testing offers numerous benefits for children, the most significant of which may be the potential for a diagnosis that is treatable and/or reveals guidance for medical screening and management that would not otherwise have been offered. The AMA Code of Medical Ethics opinion guidelines encourage genetic testing for a child when *a child is at risk for a condition for which effective measures to treat or ameliorate it are available*. Genetic testing in children is often pursued based on the assessment that the benefits of testing outweigh any burdens or risks. Depending on the age of the child, this assessment is often done by the provider in conjunction with the guardian.

It is natural to assume that most parents/guardians have their children's best interests in mind, but it is important to remember the complexities inherent in genetic testing and the potential harm that a test result may have on a child, parent, or other family member. The genetic counselor's role is important in helping families and providers to discuss and address the implications of what can be genuine but competing motivations for testing to ensure that the decision to test is indeed an appropriate one (Menzel and Madrigal 2022).

Genetic counselors have an extra responsibility when considering the testing of a minor to ensure that both the guardian and minor have a thorough and age-appropriate understanding of the benefits and potential current and future burdens to

DOI: 10.1201/9781003397847-10

Table 10.1   Potential Benefits and Potential Risks/Burdens of Genetic Testing for Minors

BENEFITS	RISKS OR BURDENS
Medical diagnosis with actionable treatment and/or screening	Psychological consequences of "no answer" and disappointment in continuation of diagnostic journey
Ending the diagnostic journey (benefit to family as well)	Diagnosis may unearth additional medical concerns, guilt, or fear
A genetic diagnosis may alleviate guilt or worry from the family that they did something wrong	Incidental findings that may be unclear or adult onset and therefore psychologically burdensome
Allows for more informed choices and planning in the future	Potential for discrimination concerns as an adult: life or health insurance, employment barriers, social concerns
Validates autonomy for minors involved in assent process	May violate child's right to an open future
Allows for additional support services/resources	Boxes child into a group or diagnosis they may not like

the child. Table 10.1 lays out some of the benefits and risks of genetic testing in minors for families to consider (Fenwick 2010).

The Right to an Open Future

Philosopher Joel Feinberg originally coined the concept of a child's "right to an open future," stating that every child is a future adult and that parents/guardians have a duty to protect each future adult's right to autonomy in their future choices (Feinberg 1992). In the context of genetic testing for minors, this suggests that it is a parent's responsibility to at the least consider how the choices they make now may limit or infringe upon the autonomy of their child at a future time (see Table 10.1 for potential burdens) (Garrett et al. 2019). One should consider, for example, how an adult who received a genetic diagnosis as a child may feel that the option to make an informed choice regarding knowledge about their own genetic information had been taken away.

There is consensus that routine carrier screening and predictive genetic testing for adult-onset disorders should not be offered to children in most circumstances in support of the right-to-an-open-future concept. The best interest principle is an ethical framework used in the publication of the 2013 American Academy of Pediatrics (AAP) and American College of Medical Genetics (ACMG) joint policy statement on genetic testing in children, which recommends against predictive genetic testing unless interventions in childhood are likely to decrease morbidity and mortality, with few valid exceptions (Fallot and Katz 2013).

Obtaining Informed Consent or Assent

The "informed consent" process for adults has three main elements: (1) disclosure of information to patients and their surrogates, (2) assessment of patient and surrogate understanding and capacity of decision-making, and (3) obtaining informed consent before any testing or treatment. Older children and adolescents should be informed about and given the option of participation in conversations about genetic testing; they may have the capacity for decision-making and therefore may be able to participate in the informed consent process. This should be assessed and addressed on a case-by-case basis (Wilfond and Diekema 2012).

Because a young child does not have the capacity to consent, the goal is to obtain assent rather that informed consent. Assent is defined as the expression of understanding and willingness to participate. The role of the parent and healthcare provider in this process is essential and should consider the child's understanding, reasoning, and interest in participation (Katz and Webb 2016). If, after the consent/assent process, a child declines genetic testing, their voice should be respected and alternative options/delay in testing should be considered. It would be a rare circumstance in which a child's dissent should be overridden by their guardian(s), and such a case would be an appropriate one for discussion at a hospital ethics committee (Farber and Blustein 2021).

NSGC's most recent (2018) position statement on genetic testing of minors for adult-onset conditions states that *The decision for a minor to undergo genetic testing that could identify variants for adult-onset conditions either specifically or secondarily (e.g. through genomic sequencing) should be made cautiously, and whenever possible, with appropriate assent of the minor (see Chapter 23).*

Results Disclosure and Follow-Up

As is evident in the advancements in genetic testing in just over the last 50 years, the meaning and interpretation of genetic test results is constantly evolving. Ensuring that the adults who had genetic testing as children continue to have their results protected, have access to reinterpretation of their results, and are offered the opportunity for conversations with genetic providers is essential in reenforcing an ethical approach to genetic testing for children.

Processes for test result disclosure and follow-up should be well defined when performing genetic testing on minors. Children and adults will process results differently, and there should be a support system with resources in place to help children and families navigate this information. Patient support groups can be especially useful for those children and families receiving a new diagnosis (Crellin et al. 2023). As results are reclassified and new genetic information emerges, adults who had testing as children should have the same access to this new information as adult patients.

When possible, a child should be included in results-disclosure conversations, and it is important to follow best practices in these conversations; most often, a multidisciplinary approach is best. Colleagues such as child life specialists, child psychologists, chaplains, and social workers are important resources, and there are also many helpful online tools and resources for families and genetic counselors that can help with these discussions. Guidelines for addressing scenarios in which parents may request that their children not be informed of results should be well thought out with context and respect for each individual and family situation at the forefront. When possible, family-centered care should be weighed and balanced with the respect for the child's autonomy.

The NSGC (2018) position statement on genetic testing of minors for adult-onset conditions states that *If a minor undergoes testing and results are not disclosed to the child, the health care provider should discuss strategies with the parents/guardian for sharing the results as he/she develops capacity or at the age of capacity. As always, each family and case is unique, and processes and recommendations may be guided differently for children and adults with intellectual disabilities (see Chapter 17).*

Case Study

Olivia is a 11-year-old girl with mild developmental delay and hearing loss. She last had targeted genetic testing when she was 4 years old, which was normal, and at her appointment this year, her geneticist briefly mentions the option of whole-exome sequencing (WES) to Olivia and her parents.

Olivia's parents learn that their insurance will cover the testing and schedule an appointment for Olivia and them to meet with a genetic counselor to review the benefits, limitations, and potential burdens of the testing. The day of the appointment, Olivia is not feeling well. The family has been waiting 6 months for this appointment and don't want to miss it, so her parents leave Olivia with her grandmother so that they may go and meet with the genetic counselor. At the end of that visit, her parents sign the consent forms, and the genetic counselor gives them a lab slip for them to take Olivia to the lab when she feels better to get her blood drawn. A follow-up appointment is scheduled for 3 months to review results.

Three months later, the family returns for the WES results. The genetic counselor sits down with the three of them and reviews the results, which show that Olivia has two mutations in the *USH2* gene, consistent with a diagnosis of Usher syndrome type II, an autosomal recessive genetic disorder characterized by progressive hearing loss and vision loss (typical vision loss onset in late adolescence or early adulthood).

Olivia is shocked. When she went to have her blood drawn, her parents had told her that the genetic test was intended to uncover the reason for her learning disabilities and hearing loss. She was hoping that the results would help to uncover why school was so hard for her and maybe even lead her to resources to help her in this area. Now, the genetic counselor was telling her that the learning differences weren't necessarily related to the diagnosis of Usher syndrome and that she was likely going to start losing her vision in her teen years *and* continue to lose her hearing! She had not realized that the test results had the potential to uncover an additional worry/concern for her. Olivia breaks down crying and runs out of the room. The genetic counselor is stunned. Olivia's father runs after Olivia, and her mother turns to the genetic counselor and says, "We never should have done this testing without including her in the conversation. We thought we understood the potential benefits and burdens and how to weight those, but we should have made sure that Olivia did as well. Now, she is crushed by her diagnosis, angry with us, and will never trust us or the medical system again."

KEY POINT SUMMARY

- The genetic counselor plays a key role within a multidisciplinary team in assessing the appropriateness of genetic testing and highlighting the potential benefits and burdens of genetic testing that are unique to minors.
- Children should be included in age-appropriate pre- and posttest counseling conversations.
- The negative aspects of impinging upon the future choice of individuals when testing minors should be acknowledged.
- The consent/assent process should include professionals who are familiar with the pediatric population and should be evaluated on a case-by-case basis.
- Special attention should be paid to how children will/do receive access to and follow-up for genetic test results as adolescents and adults.
- Consideration should be given to the potential future harms that any genetic testing may have on a child, and support resources should be made available to children and their families.

References

AMA Code of Medical Ethics. *Opinion 2.2.5: Genetic Testing of Children [Internet]*. https://code-medical-ethics.ama-assn.org/sites/amacoedb/files/2022-08/2.2.5.pdf

Crellin E et al. What matters to parents? A scoping review of parents' service experiences and needs regarding genetic testing for rare diseases. *Eur J Hum Genet*. 2023;31:869–878.

Fallot M, Katz A. Ethical and policy issues in genetic testing and screening of children. *Pediatrics*. 2013;131(3):620–622.

Farber Post L, Blustein J. *Handbook for Health Care Ethics Committees*. Johns Hopkins University Press, 2021.

Feinberg J. The child's right to an open future. In: Feinberg J, ed., *Freedom and Fulfillment: Philosophical Essays*. Princeton University Press, 1992:76–97.

Fenwick J. Are guidelines for genetic testing of children necessary? *Fam Cancer*. 2010;9:23–25.

Garrett J et al. Rethinking the "open future" argument against predictive genetic testing of children. *Genet Med*. 2019;21(10):2190–2198.

Katz A, Webb S, AAP Committee on Bioethics. Informed consent in decision making in pediatric practice. *Pediatrics*. 2016;138(2).

Menzel M, Madrigal VN. Genetic testing and screening of children. In: Nortje NN, Bester JC, eds., *Pediatric Ethics: Theory and Practice*. Springer, 2022:313–328.

Moore A, Richer J. Genetic testing and screening in children: Position statement. *Paediatr Child Health*. 2022;27(4):243–247.

National Society of Genetic Counselors. *Genetic Testing of Minors for Adult-Onset Conditions [Internet]*, 2018. ww.nsgc.org/POLICY/Position-Statements/Position-Statements/Post/genetic-testing-of-minors-for-adult-onset-conditions

Wilfond BS, Diekema DS. Engaging children in genomics research: Decoding the meaning of assent in research. *Genet Med*. 2012;14:437–443.

11

Obtaining Consent in Acute Settings

MICHELE DISCO

Introduction

Increasingly, genetic counselors are the specialists responding to genetic consultation requests from providers in pediatric or adult intensive care units. Results may assist providers in addressing active medical issues, ideally before a patient leaves the hospital. The basic skills of a genetic counselor are similar in both outpatient and inpatient settings. However, the immediate concerns of the family and the consenting process can be dramatically different in intensive care than in a planned visit.

This chapter addresses consenting in acute settings by a genetics professional, typically a genetic counselor. The nurses, residents, and hospitalists assigned to care for inpatients during the stay are referred to as the "floor team." If over 18, the individual consents for themselves. If the patient is a child, their parents will consent for them. I have referred to "families" as those who give permission for genetic testing to cover both settings. The challenge is not just obtaining signed consent but making the bidirectional discussion of risks, benefits, and family priorities a positive and productive experience.

Challenges and Strategies

Loss of Control/Unpredictability

Reducing unpredictability helps establish trust, which is important for this voluntary process. Just as families consent for genetic testing, they need to first consent to an assessment for appropriate testing. As the established contacts, the floor team first broaches the possibility of a genetic evaluation, and if the family agrees, they request a consultation. Reaching the family by phone before arriving at bedside grants them a degree of control. For the genetic counselors, knowing if the medical historian or consenting individual is at bedside is helpful before making the trip. If they are not at bedside, intake information can be taken by phone. At minimum, if the advance phone call was unanswered, the genetics staff can state they attempted to phone in advance.

 DOI: 10.1201/9781003397847-11

Clear and immediate contracting is vital, including describing the flow and time frame of a consultation, review of the record, the role of the geneticist or genetic counselor, and the requirement for consent for any genetic testing. Use names with roles and give business cards. Being clear and direct, no matter the family's comprehension level, is helpful to a sick individual or an anxious family's understanding. Tell them the costs, if through insurance or the institution, before reviewing the fine print of consent. The financial ramifications of the hospital bill and absence from work are present for families and may derail their ability to listen to complicated information.

Another frequent concern for families is whether testing requires a blood draw and whether parent samples are also needed. Describing how the sample is obtained is important to reducing the unknown.

Good communication between families and medical staff has been shown to reduce parental stress and anxiety. Additionally, the medical team should have the same "story" about genetic testing. Once the genetics team has left, the family may well be asking the bedside nurse any outstanding questions. Making sure the floor team accurately understands the sample needs will reduce the conflicting information families may receive.

Understanding: Why Genetic Testing and Why Now? Setting Expectations

What are the goals of genetic testing in the acute setting? Patients and parents are faced with the confounding combination of highly technical information and many "maybes." Maybe the results will help; maybe they will be another dead end in the search to heal their family member. Some patients will agree to any testing their primary team recommends; others are more skeptical. Clearly stating the purpose of a genetic test is essential, and the purpose should be the same if the family asks another provider.

Generally, the primary purpose of inpatient testing is to guide management of the current hospitalization or longer-term care of the precipitating problem. For instance, if seizures are caused by a genetic finding of Dravet syndrome, certain medications are more effective, while others can exacerbate seizures. Establishing the likelihood of a positive result sets expectations for the family and for the care team. Studies have shown that parents overestimate the chances of receiving a clear diagnostic outcome from genetic testing and overestimate the effect of a positive result on medication choice or the ability to "cure" the condition. The GC does not have to quote an exact percentage of positives, which varies based on the patient's age, family history, range of affected systems, and severity of symptoms. Sometimes, care changes following a positive result are subtle, or GCs cannot say *a priori* that the genetic result will affect medical care. Be clear: A positive result *may* help guide future care. If possible, describe exactly how. Simply stating "most of the time, testing is negative" can be helpful. Describing the percentage of new variants compared to familial variants can be helpful. The GC should be transparent and give a realistic range so families can base their expectations accordingly.

Conversely, a negative result can reduce uncertainty for the floor team sorting through their differential diagnosis, rule out known genetic causes, or lead the geneticist to recommend further testing. Returning the locus of control to the parents, the result will give the family more information about how to care for their loved one.

If genetic testing will not assist in treatment or is not for an acute condition, deferring to an outpatient appointment is reasonable. For instance, an acute consult to rule out neurofibromatosis type 1 due to multiple café-au-lait spots and autism in a patient hospitalized for infectious disease should be deferred. In contrast to the outpatient setting, recurrence risks for a known condition in future children are not a primary inpatient concern and not a reason for inpatient testing. Recurrence risks are best addressed by reproductive genetic counselors at a set appointment.

Patients may be accustomed to test results coming back within days or even later the same day. Discuss the length of time that is needed to receive a genetic result (turnaround time, or TAT) to set an appropriate expectation. Surprisingly, some people are under the impression they will need to stay in the hospital until a genetic result is returned. Describe how they will receive results, including that they will be notified of negative results. Reiterating that the patient has a medical issue and will be cared for based on symptoms while results are pending can be reassuring.

Timeliness

In most inpatient consultations, the order must be honored and completed within 24 hours. Knowing there are generally long TATs, a floor team may be interested in sending genetic testing as soon as possible to assist with a differential diagnosis. The genetics team may also be interested in completing the case as quickly as possible. However, families are asked to make a complicated decision for which time to comprehend the benefits and limitations or the time to consider the counsel of other family or community is important. The GC must balance the need for speed with the family's need to understand testing and feel confident with a choice to proceed.

Again, clarity in describing the purpose of the test is essential; so is insisting to the floor team that a family needs more time. Some families will benefit from a second or third visit or a phone call to an absent parent. Having printed or video materials available allows for review, different learning styles, and sharing among family who may not have been present originally. While some will want testing as soon as possible, a family that feels rushed by genetics or the floor team may regret their choice. A day more before testing is sent is often time well invested in a family's informed decision.

In the rush, important caveats still need to be conveyed. For some patients, results may affect the surgical or transplant options offered. A microarray can show homozygosity, indicating a blood relationship between the mother and father. If trio testing has been offered, mis-attributed parentage (or a rare chimera) may be evident in the results.

Occasionally, a family will decline genetic testing. Probing as to why they are declining can help with honest misunderstandings but also in supporting the family's decision when the requesting care team is eager. Recognizing a family's right to decline and remaining available respectfully leaves the option of genetic testing open.

Adults without Capacity

When seeking consent for adult patients without capacity in an inpatient setting, genetic counselors must navigate complex ethical and procedural considerations. These include assessing the patient's prognosis, the expected duration of incapacity, and the potential benefits of testing for both the patient and their family. In cases in which the incapacity is temporary, deferring genetic testing until the patient can provide informed consent themselves may be appropriate to ensure autonomy is upheld. Conversely, when recovery is uncertain or tenuous, involving family members or next of kin to provide consent – while considering their relationship to the patient and the potential utility of the results – may be justified. Additionally, the urgency of the genetic information for medical decision-making or familial risk assessment must be carefully weighed. Collaborating with the care team is essential. Consider seeking a consultation with the hospital's ethics board to ensure decisions respect the patient's rights, align with medical and ethical standards, and balance the needs of the patient and their family.

Case Study

Working with the following family in the neonatal intensive care unit (NICU) illustrates many of the points in this chapter.

WD, a 9-day-old baby boy born at 35 weeks by Caesarean section, was transferred to our hospital due to concerns for a metabolic condition. His birthweight was 2.9 kg. He had high hematocrit and lactic acidosis with prenatally recognized biventricular hypertrophy and dilated bowel loops. He was intubated for respiratory distress.

WD's mother had normal noninvasive genetic screening (NIPS) during pregnancy. No other genetic testing had been performed. Family history was significant for the loss of a sister at 15 days old with similar symptoms, including hypertrophic cardiomyopathy. Exome sequencing sent for his sister was negative. Rapid genome sequencing for the newborn was proposed to the family at the previous hospital, but they were undecided, and no samples were sent. Parents were also given the option for a targeted cardiomyopathy panel, but they did not see the benefit for their son.

Meanwhile, metabolic evaluations did not indicate a likely disorder and WD's newborn screening was normal. The geneticist at our hospital agreed that rapid genome sequencing (rGS) with mitochondrial sequencing would be the best test, considering the sibling's negative exome sequencing result, WD's symptoms, and his critical status.

Initially, the family was confused about genetic testing and how it might help WD. The mother was frustrated that she didn't understand the testing and felt like it was being pushed to her without a clear benefit for her child. She became angry that doctors at both hospitals were not communicating with her – "They don't explain anything, and I'm his mother."

Taking a step back when faced with anger is useful. The team likely felt they were communicating appropriately. This family is grieving a previous child while seeing a similar situation emerge for their newborn. Transferring to a hospital farther from home and managing extended family added to the stress they experienced. Medical teams were continuously analyzing, checking lab results, carefully escalating or deescalating as the patient responded, and ordering new tests to help them understand. For the family, uncertainty in the experts they needed to trust compounded their own. In training as a genetic counselor, we learn ways to understand the source of a parent's anger – and yet there is rarely a quiet space or stretch of time to explore the source of emotions in a busy NICU when the goal is to treat a critically ill child.

The genetics team broke down the steps of what the test does and how results might be helpful for their child. The explanations were concise, centered on the child. Rather than stating that results will help understand "why," Genetics explained that if a result is positive, "we look at other children who have the same genetic change and see how we can use information about them to help your child." They were given time to consider. After 2 days of deliberation and negative metabolic evaluation, the parents decided to go ahead with rGS and mitochondrial sequencing. The 2 days of delay may have been difficult for the anxious floor team, but they were important to the family processing this information. The parents were aware that their daughter's previous negative test reduced the chance of a positive result for WD and that we would have verbal results for this test in 7 days.

Genetics contacted the parents often with updates and an opportunity to ask questions in an effort to ameliorate their communication concerns. Trust and open communication became especially important when there was a brief lab delay in getting rapid results due to technical issues with the mother's sample.

Both rGS and mitochondrial sequencing came back negative. With worsening symptoms over the following weeks, the family decided to focus on palliation and stop intensive life-support measures. WD passed away at 35 days, in the arms of his parents.

Stress in the ICU affects genetic counselors and their medical colleagues, not just the family. Process groups, post-mortem meetings or speaking to Spiritual Care can be resources in a GC's self-care toolbox. Taking care of GCs in acute care is necessary to continuing this important work.

KEY POINT SUMMARY

- People who are hospitalized are in a time of acute stress.
- Informed decision-making remains important in this difficult setting.
- Genetics professionals can reduce uncertainty and the information load that accompanies genetic test consenting.
- Define how genetic testing will help in the patient's care in the short and long term.
- Use direct and clear language, with understandable terms.
- Consider an ethics consultation when trying to coordinate testing for an adult patient without capacity to provide consent.

Bibliography

Alzawad Z et al. Parents' challenges beyond the pediatric intensive care unit: Fraying at the seams while balancing between two worlds, home and hospital. *Children*. 2022;9:267.

Diamonstein, C. Factors complicating the informed consent process for whole exome sequencing in neonatal and pediatric intensive care units. *J Genet Counsel*. 2019:256–262.

Hill M et al. Delivering genome sequencing for rapid genetic diagnosis in critically ill children: Parent and professional views, experiences and challenges. *Eur J Hum Genet*. 2020;28(11):1529–1540.

Jarvis JM et al. Supporting families during pediatric critical illness: Opportunities identified in a multicenter, qualitative study. *J Child Healthcare*. 2023:1–13.

Lynch F et al. Parents' experiences of decision making for rapid genomic sequencing in intensive care. *Eur J Hum Genet*. 2021;29(12):1804–1810.

Roberts JS et al. Patient understanding of, satisfaction with, and perceived utility of whole-genome sequencing: Findings from the MedSeq project. *Genet Med*. 2018;20:1069–1076.

Walter JK et al. Parental communication satisfaction with the clinical team in the paediatric cardiac ICU. *Cardiol Young*. 2024;34(2):282–290.

Ethical Issues with Obtaining Consent for Predictive Genetic Testing

JILL S. GOLDMAN

Introduction

Knowing one's future and whether someone will die young or old has been a timeless concern. Prediction of one's genetic future began with the linkage of Huntington's disease (HD) in 1986 and then direct gene testing following the discovery of the *HTT* gene in 1993. In expectation of these discoveries, ethicists, scientists, clinicians, and families worried about the implications of testing at-risk individuals, fearing adverse outcomes such as suicide or severe depression. This led to the formation of HD predictive testing guidelines that established safety nets including genetic counseling and neurological and psychiatric evaluations, staggered appointments, age limits for testing, and specifications on informed consent (Goldman, 2020). As genetic testing became routine in healthcare and studies found a low incidence of adverse outcomes, guidelines were modified. Predictive genetic testing is now pervasive for cancer and cardiology, where genetic results can lead to medical interventions. Predictive genetic testing presents many ethical issues including informed consent because of the implications of results on medical management, clinical trial candidacy, significance for other family members, reproductive choices, and psychological effects. The web of complicated outcomes is particularly pertinent to neurodegenerative diseases for which there are presently no medical interventions. This chapter will examine these issues.

Challenges and Strategies

Informed Consent in the Presence of Cognitive or Psychiatric Symptoms

The term "predictive testing" implies that the person to be tested is asymptomatic of the disease for which they are testing. However, in many neurodegenerative conditions, both cognitive and psychiatric symptoms can exist long before diagnosis. This is especially true for HD and frontotemporal dementia (FTD), where many individuals can have symptoms of inappropriate behavior and poor decision-making many years before diagnosis. Similarly, people can have early cognitive symptoms impairing their ability to analyze or fully remember details of problems. When seeing people for

 DOI: 10.1201/9781003397847-12

predictive testing of these diseases, genetic counselors must be aware of the possibility of early symptoms. Additionally, at-risk individuals without early symptoms can demonstrate significant depression or anxiety due to their risk or for other reasons. Certain guidelines can help prevent inappropriate testing. Having an informant or support person attend the session with the at-risk individual can clarify whether the person has any psychiatric or cognitive changes. Requiring a neurological or psychiatric evaluation prior to testing can also be helpful. With the obviously affected individual, a physician can give a diagnosis so that the person can hear that they are already affected and decide on testing based on that information. For the person with more subtle cognitive symptoms, a physician can evaluate their competency to consent as well as their risk for psychological distress. For the client with a strong history of depression or anxiety who is still experiencing symptoms, a psychiatric evaluation prior to testing is warranted. If the person is in therapy currently, the genetic counselor can ask for permission to consult with the therapist.

Informed Consent When Testing Will Reveal Another Family Member's Genetic Status

Predictive genetic testing presents an ethical dilemma when the genetic status of the individual being tested will reveal the genetic status of another family member, as in the case of an identical twin or when an at-risk parent has chosen not to test (Stark et al. 2016). Examining these situations in pretest counseling is extremely important for a successful outcome. The counselor should try to understand whether the client has discussed genetic testing with the at-risk family members and if not, why not. Often, the answer is that they do not want to raise anxiety necessarily or that they already know that their family member does not want to be tested. The client may be willing to have a hypothetical conversation with their family about the client's possible test so that the family members can say, "If you do it, don't tell me," or "I would want to know your results." The client should be reminded that it is easier to have this discussion prior to receiving results. If the client says that they have no intention of sharing the results, the counselor should ask whether they can really keep them a secret and explore the duty to warn and the concept of the right to know or not know. The counselor may have been through these scenarios before and may choose to share problematic outcomes such as a family member who overheard results and reacted with tremendous anger at not being warned. The genetic counselor can only raise these issues. In the long run, the client must make their own decision both about informing family members and about testing.

Informed Consent in the Absence of a Significant Other or a Support Person

In most areas of genetic counseling, clients routinely go through the testing process alone. However, people undergoing predictive testing for a neurodegenerative condition are strongly encouraged to bring their significant other or a support person to both the pretest and disclosure sessions. Attending genetic counseling with another individual (such as a partner) allows the client to have someone else with whom they can discuss the information to help make a testing decision. It also allows the counselor to gain perspective on how the client will cope with potentially life-changing information. The counselor can explore how the partner would react to a pathogenic result and how supportive they would be of the client. When a couple disagrees on testing or how they would cope with the outcome, the genetic counselor should recommend postponing testing until they can come to a consensus. Referral for therapy is often helpful.

Some individuals insist on going through the testing process alone (Zimmermann et al. 2021). The genetic counselor needs to examine reasons behind this decision and the extent of the person's support system. If doubt exists about the client's ability to cope with results because of a lack of support, referral to a therapist becomes very important. Having a psychiatrist/psychologist/social worker as part of the clinical team is an advantage; however, the counselor can ask that the client meet with an outside therapist who would then be allowed to report to the counselor with a recommendation whether to proceed with testing. Although this strategy reduces autonomy, it increases nonmaleficence by protecting the client and the counselor from a potentially adverse outcome.

Informed Consent for Genetic Testing of Minors for Adult-Onset Disease

Long-standing guidelines discourage the genetic testing of minors for adult-onset disease for which there is no early intervention (NSGC 2018). This is especially true for neurodegenerative diseases. The autonomy of the minor is the first point of consideration when other family members are pushing testing. Yet guidelines recognize that circumstances exist when the minors themselves are requesting testing with or without the inclusion of their parent, such as when the minor is pregnant (emancipated minor) and when the minor is requesting testing to help clarify their future. These situations raise ethical dilemmas for genetic counselors.

The revised HD international guidelines (2013) recommend that testing be discouraged for anyone under the age of 18 but that any minor should receive genetic counseling when requested. Many HD testing centers feel that even at 18, individuals may not fully appreciate the consequences of genetic testing. The genetic counselor's task in these situations is to provide full information on the genetics of the condition and the unpredictability of age of onset and specific symptoms. In HD, for instance, the at-risk individual may not fully appreciate anticipation and the fact that they might be affected at an earlier age than their parent. On the flip side, they may not realize that if found to be a carrier, their symptoms could differ significantly from those of their parent. As such, genetic testing may not end the uncertainty. Additionally, if testing is being used to determine their life path, they may not consider possible future prevention/treatment in their decisions. Minors and young adults may not appreciate the possibility of future discrimination. Lastly, the psychological stability of minors and young adults must be carefully assessed. Retrospective reports from this group indicate mixed outcomes, with some people coping well but others regretting their choices.

However, there are some very mature 17 and 18 year olds who fully understand the implications of genetic testing for themselves and their families. They may feel the need to test to plan their immediate futures such as choice of college or to alleviate the uncertainty that may be causing anxiety. The genetic counselor can help these individuals examine their motivation for testing and why it cannot wait for a few years. If the counselor feels that the reasons are valid, that they have a supportive network around them, and that the individual is psychologically stable, testing may be reasonable. The counselor should discuss the case with the HD team and require a psychological evaluation. As discussed in the 2013 EHDN guidelines, on a case-by-case basis, certain minors can be tested.

Informed Consent for Genetic Testing of People for Clinical Trial Participation

The availability of clinical trials has produced another ethical issue for genetic counselors (Uhlmann and Roberts 2018). Some individuals who never wished to learn their genetic status will decide to do so when a positive test might make them eligible for a trial. Giving informed consent under these circumstances means that the client must understand what the trial involves, the eligibility criteria, and the uncertainty about success. The genetic counselor must make sure that their client realizes that they might not be accepted into the trial and that the trial could be stopped. Therefore, the client must be comfortable knowing their genetic status regardless of the trial. The genetic counselor should determine whether there is pressure to test from either the medical team or the family. If present, the counselor should have a discussion with the medical team and/or family about the psychological consequences and the limitations of testing for clinical trial participation.

Informed Consent in the Presence of Family Coercion

Many people delay testing until their children are in significant relationships. At that point, they may feel obliged to have testing to give their children information. This reason for testing can produce substantial anxiety about their own risk, how to inform their children, and their children's risk. Pressure to test may be exerted by the not-at-risk spouse or by the children themselves. The role of the genetic counselor in these situations is to help the at-risk individual realistically determine how a positive test would impact their life (the onset could be soon) and plan how and when to discuss testing with their children. The genetic counselor must offer the right not to know despite the pressure being put on the client. The following case study illustrates the complexity of this situation.

Case Study

Carl and Joanne had visited the HD Center several times over the past decade because his paternal uncle had died of HD in his late 60s. Carl's father had three other younger siblings who were unaffected. Carl's father died of an aneurysm at age 54 without any HD symptoms. Carl's paternal grandfather died of pneumonia at 85 and was "a little shaky." His paternal grandmother died of kidney failure at 89. Carl was 64 at the current visit. Carl and Joanne had a married daughter who had two children and a newly married son.

Carl and Joanne's first visit was primarily for information. Neither of them really wanted to know about Carl's status because he was fine, and their daughter had chronic depression, so they did not want to raise any concerns. Their second visit came following a family wedding at which they learned that their 45-year-old nephew was affected. This information raised substantial anxiety for the couple. Their daughter now had children and would not be having any more. However, their son was getting married. Although Carl and Joanne felt that testing probably was not needed because Carl was already older than his uncle, they wanted reassurance.

The genetic counselor validated their concerns but reminded them that Carl's risk was uncertain because of the reduced penetrance range of HD where someone can be an asymptomatic carrier and transmit the gene. She encouraged them to speak with their children before Carl decided on testing to give them the right to know or not know their father's status. However, they didn't want to ruin their son's upcoming wedding and were not going to tell their daughter. After his psychiatric and neurological evaluations, Carl scheduled the genetic test but postponed it because of COVID.

The next appointment came after their son's wedding. It was clear that Carl did not want testing but felt obliged to test before their son had children. Again, the counselor discussed communicating with their son. If Carl didn't want to test, his son could test instead. Following another denial, testing was ordered. Results revealed that Carl had 38 CAG repeats (reduced penetrance range). The couple said they would inform their son, but by the time they did, their son and daughter-in-law were pregnant. Upon finally hearing Carl's results, their son was furious that he had not been informed years before about Carl's risk. The son pursued his own testing, which resulted in the same 38 CAG repeats. The fetus was found to be normal on prenatal testing. In summary, the family relationship was changed indefinitely.

This case demonstrated how genetic counselors may be unable to establish the ideal situation for genetic testing. The client may make decisions based on emotion that could backfire. The counselor should encourage family discussion, offer a family meeting, or offer to test another family member, but in the end, they can only be supportive (Nurmi et al. 2020).

KEY POINT SUMMARY

- Predictive testing can reveal the status of someone else who does not want to know.
- A support person is beneficial.
- Predictive testing for clinical trial participation may not be appropriate.
- Predictive testing of minors should be evaluated carefully.
- Lack of family communication can negatively impact the predictive testing process.

References

Goldman JS. Predictive genetic counseling for neurodegenerative diseases: Past, present, and future. *Cold Spring Harb Perspect Med.* 2020;10(7):a036525.

Huntington Disease Society of America. *Genetic Testing Protocol for Huntington's Disease [Internet]*, 2016. http://hdsa.org/wp-content/uploads/2015/02/HDSA-Gen-Testing-Protocol-for-HD.pdf

MacLeod R et al. Editorial committee and working group 'genetic testing counselling' of the European Huntington Disease Network. Recommendations for the predictive genetic test in Huntington's disease. *Clin Genet.* 2013;83(3):221–231.

National Society of Genetic Counselors. *Genetic Testing of Minors for Adult-Onset Conditions [Internet]*, 2018. www.nsgc.org/POLICY/Position-Statements/Position-Statements/Post/genetic-testing-of-minors-for-adult-onset-conditions

Nurmi SM et al. The ethical implications of genetic testing in neurodegenerative diseases: A systematic review. *Scand J Caring Sci.* 2020;35(4):1057–1074.

Roberts JS et al. Genetic testing for neurodegenerative diseases: Ethical and health communication challenges. *Neurobiol Dis.* 2020;141:104871.

Stark Z et al. Predictive genetic testing for neurodegenerative conditions: How should conflicting interests within families be managed? *J Med Ethics.* 2016;42(10):640–642.

Uhlmann WR, Roberts JS. Ethical issues in neurogenetics. In: Geschwind DH, Paulson HL, Klein C, eds., *Handbook of Clinical Neurology.* Elsevier, 2018;147:23–36.

Zimmermann BM et al. Autonomy and social influence in predictive genetic testing decision-making: A qualitative interview study. *Bioethics.* 2021;35(2):199–206.

13

EMERGING SPECIALTIES IN GENETIC COUNSELING

A Path towards the Future of Genetic Counseling

NATALIE VENA

Introduction

Advancements in understanding how genetic variants modify disease risk, aid in diagnoses, and inform clinical management have led to a dramatic increase in the application and utilization of genetic testing and related services across medicine. As a result, the uptake of genomic services, including genetic testing and counseling, within medical specialty areas has significantly increased over the last decade. The growing demand for genomic services for patients and their families necessitates the ongoing collaboration between genetic counselors and nongenetic medical providers across medical disciplines and has given rise to emerging genetic specialties in medicine. Areas such as cardiology and neurology were among the first in medicine to recognize the importance and necessity of specialized genetics clinics. However, with the rapid advancement of molecular diagnostics and the increasing understanding of the genetic basis of diseases, genomic services are being utilized in new areas of medicine, and specialty genetics clinics, such as nephrology, ophthalmology, and psychiatry, are on the rise. While making up less than 10% of the overall genetic counseling workforce, these specialty areas (i.e., those other than adult cancer, prenatal, and pediatrics) represent a growing and expanding area of practice, with over 16 areas of direct patient care positions reported on the 2023 National Society of Genetic Counselors (NSGC) Professional Status Survey. This rapid expansion and development of emerging genetic specialists have ushered in a new set of challenges and considerations for the field of genetic counseling as specialty areas strive to stay abreast of the growing body of genetic knowledge.

This chapter explores the emergence of specialty areas in genetic counseling practices, highlights some practical considerations for establishing emerging specialty genetic clinics, and examines the utility of these clinics in the field of genetics and patient care.

DOI: 10.1201/9781003397847-13

Challenges and Strategies

The Emergence of the Specialty Genetic Clinic in Medicine

The field of clinical genetics has been grappling with a shortage of qualified genetics healthcare professionals, including medical geneticists and genetic counselors, for the past 20 years despite the increased utilization of genomic services in medicine. The prevailing clinical delivery model is a genetics-led program, with 13 U.S.-based programs providing all genetic counseling and care within general medical genetics settings. However, these programs are impacted by a workforce shortage, long appointment wait times, and geographical limitations. The increased application of genetics across healthcare, combined with a shrinking workforce, has led to a higher demand for genomic services in all areas of medicine. The utilization of telemedicine, accelerated by the COVID-19 pandemic, has improved wait times and patient satisfaction and increased access to genomic services. However, traditional service delivery models are still predominantly used and have not been able to keep up with the growing needs of the field. As the application of genetics across medical specialties continues to grow, innovative service delivery models are needed to improve patient access and support the increased utilization of genomic services.

Innovative and efficient delivery models are necessary to meet the growing demand for genomic services in medicine. One approach to meet this increasing need is to maximize the efficiency of the existing genetics workforce by creating genetics clinics within medical specialties across healthcare. In these specialty genetics clinics, a multidisciplinary approach to care is utilized, in which a nongenetics medical provider is paired with a genetics professional to facilitate the provision of genetics services within their specific medical specialty and patient population. While a multidisciplinary approach to genomics services is not novel, it has gained renewed interest in recent years. This model now represents the second-most common genomic service delivery model, accounting for nearly 55 programs worldwide. This approach is well utilized and has proven successful in areas such as cancer genetics and cardiology, resulting in several benefits, such as shorter wait times, increased access, and uptake of genomic services. As the collaboration between nongenetic and genetic providers spreads to other areas of medicine and becomes mainstream, genetic counselors are uniquely positioned to utilize their professional skill set to facilitate the development and growth of these specialty clinics.

While these nontraditional delivery models have demonstrated several benefits to patient care, incorporating genetics into specialty areas of medicine is limited by nongenetic medical providers' lack of genetic knowledge. Multiple studies have found that while nongenetics medical providers recognize the advantages of genetic care and routinely engage in discussions around genetic testing, they often report a limited understanding of general genetic concepts, even within the context of their medical specialties. Moreover, even when genetics is discussed, nongenetics providers report limited awareness of relevant genetic tests, low confidence in selecting appropriate testing, and difficulty interpreting genetic test results. These limitations illustrate the need for a collaborative, multidisciplinary approach to genomic services and care within the medical specialty setting.

The growing recognition for improved genetics education for nongenetics providers is driving significant efforts to equip them with foundational knowledge in genetics. Significant, systemic efforts have been made to train new providers in genetics and genomics, but special considerations should also focus on those currently practicing in their specialty area. Continuing medical education (CME) programs have emerged as one of the most common settings for genetics training among physicians and, therefore, hold significant potential for educational reform. In addition, online tools and web-based curricula and programs can also improve provider knowledge of genetics but are contingent on ongoing engagement, and support from genetic providers is critical to their success. As such, genetic counselors practicing within medical specialty areas can play a vital role in educating their nongenetics colleagues. They are well positioned and suited to engage nongenetics medical providers in genetics education to promote the growth of genomic services within medical specialties. By educating healthcare providers in genomic medicine, multidisciplinary precision medicine programs reported a fivefold increase in referrals to clinical genetics and genetic specialists from 2013 to 2020, leading to improved provider education and better patient outcomes. Collectively, these efforts will continue to contribute to enhanced provider education, equipping them with a foundational knowledge of genetics and enabling them to leverage this genetic information for optimal patient outcomes.

Despite ongoing efforts to educate, keeping up with the rapidly evolving and growing field of genetics is a significant challenge for genetics providers and nongenetics providers alike. This growth is evident by the 51,803 new genetic tests introduced in the US over the past decade, representing a substantial increase from 607 tests in 2012. Therefore, continuous professional development is essential for genetic counselors to stay abreast of the latest genetic discoveries, research, and clinical recommendations. While most genetic counselors currently specialize in cancer, prenatal, or pediatrics, further specialization has emerged as the field of genetic counseling has grown. Specialized genetic counseling in areas such as psychiatric genetics has shown positive outcomes, including increased empowerment and self-efficacy for individuals with a personal history of mental illness. By focusing their skills and knowledge, genetic counselors are better equipped to manage complex presentations and provide more effective patient care when providing care in a specialty setting. As genetic counseling continues to evolve beyond its original scope of practice, it has become a broad and diverse field encompassing a wide range of clinical specialties. This evolution has led to the emergence of genetic specialty areas and the application of genetics in medical specialties, further improving patient outcomes.

The Evolving Landscape of Emerging Genetic Specialties in Medicine

Genetic testing within medical specialties and for common diseases is increasingly recognized as a critical factor in disease etiology, understanding, and management. Thus, the increasing application, availability, and affordability of genetic testing have given rise to genetic specialty areas or emerging genetic specialties. Cardiology was one of the first specialty areas to apply genetics and genomics technologies over 25 years ago, with the discovery of the first genes responsible for hypertrophic cardiomyopathy (HCM) and congenital long-QT syndrome (LQTS) in 1990 and 1995. Since then, this area of genetics has grown from monogenetic familial testing to broad, presymptomatic screening in healthy populations. Following in its footsteps, several other specialty areas for common and seemingly multifactorial or nongenetic conditions have grown tremendously. Areas such as nephrology, psychiatry, ophthalmology, hepatology, and pulmonology have all seen a tremendous increase in the application of genetics within their specialty, and precision medicine initiatives are a national initiative in medicine.

In the setting of kidney disease, genomic medicine has radically changed our understanding of the disease and downstream clinical care. Adult-onset chronic kidney disease, which affects approximately 1 in 7 adults, has been shown to have a genetic etiology in 10% to 20% of cases, and over 600 genes are noted to have a causal role in the development of the disease. Understanding the genetic etiology of kidney disease has led to a change in management in over 60% of patients with a positive result, including altered prevalence, changes in treatment, and the addition of diagnostic procedures. Similarly, the discovery of the *APOL1* high-risk genotype and the risk of kidney disease has drastically changed our understanding of the disproportionately high rates of kidney disease in populations of sub-Saharan African ancestry. Up to 13% of individuals with sub-Saharan African ancestry are predicted to have a high-risk genotype, and a high-risk genotype is associated with a three- to fivefold increased risk of developing chronic kidney disease. In addition, patients with a high-risk *APOL1* genotype progress to ESKD faster than those without a high-risk genotype, and ~40% of patients with sub-Saharan African ancestry and nondiabetic ESKD are suspected of having a high-risk genotype. The discovery of *APOL1*-mediated kidney disease has resulted in several ongoing clinical trials and advanced the field of precision medicine in nephrology. Medical specialty clinics, such as those focusing on kidney disease, highlight the benefit of extensive and comprehensive genetic care to patients in the medical specialty setting, aiding in the diagnosis, education, and research of these patients.

The identification of genetic etiologies within medical specialty fields allows for the personalized assessment of disease risk and progression, recognition of clinically related manifestations, and the assessment of disease risk in family members. When using a broad genomic approach, successful specialty genetics clinics in ophthalmology have demonstrated a positive diagnostic yield in up to 33% of patients tested and up to 6% in chronic liver disease. As such, as our understanding of the genetic etiology of diseases within medical specialty areas grows, the impact on clinical care grows as well. In current practice, specific clinical guidelines around genetic testing and clinical care related to genomic care within these areas still need to be expanded. To this end, working groups have been established in pulmonology to create guidance on genetic testing in patients with pulmonary fibrosis. Similarly, patients now find themselves eligible for gene-specific clinical trials or therapies, as evident in the field of hepatology, with over 250 clinical trials identified related to monogenic forms of liver diseases. In the near future, patients may find themselves eligible for specific medications based on their genetic etiology, as highlighted by the recent case of *APOL1*-mediated kidney disease. As genetic testing becomes more widespread across these specialty areas, the practical application of genetic testing in clinical care will continue to expand, and the benefits to patient care will be notable.

Emerging genetic specialty areas provide new and exciting opportunities for genetic counselors to collaborate with genetics and nongenetic professionals in interdisciplinary teams and draw upon their expertise. However, despite the widespread recognition of the potential value and benefits of genomic services in clinical care, multiple barriers, such as educational, institutional, and systemic limitations, prevent genetic services from being routinely adopted in medical specialties. To overcome these obstacles, various initiatives are being implemented to minimize barriers and increase genetic access by establishing emerging specialty genetics clinics. These initiatives aim to highlight the clinical expertise of genetic counselors and promote genetic testing across medical disciplines, leading to the successful integration and uptake of genetic services in medical specialties.

KEY POINT SUMMARY

- A shortage of genetics professionals and traditional service model limitations have driven the need for innovative approaches like specialty genetic clinics, which improve access and reduce wait times.
- Medical fields such as cardiology, nephrology, and hepatology increasingly use genetics to understand disease, personalize treatment, and enhance care outcomes.
- Nongenetics providers often lack the knowledge needed for effective genetic care, highlighting the critical role of genetic counselors in education and collaboration.
- These clinics improve diagnostics, enable personalized treatment plans, and provide access to clinical trials, significantly enhancing patient outcomes.
- Efforts to expand genomic services focus on reducing systemic and educational challenges, fostering broader adoption of genetic testing in medical specialties.
- Genetic counselors must stay updated on advancements in genetics to address the field's rapid growth and adapt to emerging specialty areas, ensuring effective patient care and education.

Bibliography

Andreassen OA et al. New insights from the last decade of research in psychiatric genetics: Discoveries, challenges and clinical implications. *World Psychiatry*. 2023;22(1):4–24. https://doi.org/10.1002/wps.21034

Blout Zawatsky CL et al. Workforce considerations when building a precision medicine program. *J Personalized Med*. 2022;12(11):1929. https://doi.org/10.3390/jpm12111929

Campion M et al. Genomic education for the next generation of health-care providers. *Genet Med*. 2019;21(11), 2422–2430. https://doi.org/10.1038/s41436-019-0548-4

Couser NL et al. The evolving role of genetics in ophthalmology. *Ophthal Genet*. 2021;42(2):110–113. https://doi.org/10.1080/13816810.2020.1868011

Dahl NK et al. The clinical utility of genetic testing in the diagnosis and management of adults with chronic kidney disease. *J Am Soc Nephrol*. 2023;34(12):2039–2050. https://doi.org/10.1681/ASN.0000000000000249

East KM et al. Education and training of non-genetics providers on the return of genome sequencing results in a NICU setting. *J Personalized Med*. 2023;12(3):405. https://doi.org/10.3390/jpm12030405

Elliott MD et al. Clinical and genetic characteristics of CKD patients with high-risk APOL1 genotypes. *J Am Soc Nephrol*. 2023a;34(5):909–919. https://doi.org/10.1681/ASN.0000000000000094

Elliott MD et al. Genetics of kidney disease: The unexpected role of rare disorders. *Ann Rev Med*. 2023b;74:353–367. https://doi.org/10.1146/annurev-med-042921-101813

French EL et al. Physician perception of the importance of medical genetics and genomics in medical education and clinical practice. *Med Educat Online*. 2023;28(1):2143920. https://doi.org/10.1080/10872981.2022.2143920

Gorrie A et al. Benefits and limitations of telegenetics: A literature review. *J Genet Counsel*. 2021;30(4):924–937. https://doi.org/10.1002/jgc4.1418

Haga SB et al. Development of competency-based online genomic medicine training (COGENT). *Personal Med*. 2023;20(1):55–64. https://doi.org/10.2217/pme-2022-0101

Halbisen AL, Lu CY. Trends in availability of genetic tests in the United States, 2012–2022. *J Personal Med*. 2023;13(4):638. https://doi.org/10.3390/jpm13040638

Inglis A et al. Evaluating a unique, specialist psychiatric genetic counseling clinic: Uptake and impact. *Clin Genet*. 2015;87(3):218–224. https://doi.org/10.1111/cge.12415

Jenkins BD et al. The 2019 US Medical Genetics Workforce: A focus on clinical genetics. *Genet Med*. 2021;23(8):1458–1464. https://doi.org/10.1038/s41436-021-01162-5

KDIGO Conference Participants. Genetics in chronic kidney disease: Conclusions from a Kidney Disease: Improving Global Outcomes (KDIGO) Controversies Conference. *Kidney Int*. 2022;101(6):1126–1141. https://doi.org/10.1016/j.kint.2022.03.019

Kong XF et al. The diagnostic yield of exome sequencing in liver diseases from a curated gene panel. *Scientific Rep*. 2023;13(1):21540. https://doi.org/10.1038/s41598-023-42202-1

Massingham LJ et al. Association of Professors of Human and Medical Genetics (APHMG) consensus-based update of the core competencies for undergraduate medical education in genetics and genomics. *Genet Med*. 2022;24(10):2167–2179. https://doi.org/10.1016/j.gim.2022.07.014

Morrow A et al. The design, implementation, and effectiveness of intervention strategies aimed at improving genetic referral practices: A systematic review of the literature. *Genet Med*. 2021;23(12):2239–2249. https://doi.org/10.1038/s41436-021-01272-0

National Society of Genetic Counselors. *2023 Professional Status Survey [Internet]*, 2023. www.nsgc.org/Policy-Research-and-Publications/Professional-Status-Survey

Newton CA et al. The role of genetic testing in pulmonary fibrosis: A perspective from the pulmonary fibrosis foundation genetic testing work group. *Chest*. 2022;162(2):394–405. https://doi.org/10.1016/j.chest.2022.03.023

Parekh B et al. Design and outcomes of a novel multidisciplinary ophthalmic genetics clinic. *Genes*. 2023;14(3):726. https://doi.org/10.3390/genes14030726

Pierle JM et al. Genetic service delivery models: Exploring approaches to care for families with hereditary cancer risk. *Clin J Oncol Nursing*. 2019;23(1):60–67. https://doi.org/10.1188/19.CJON.60-67

Rickman AF et al. A descriptive investigation of clinical practice models used by cardiovascular genetic counselors in North America. *J Genet Counsel*. 2023;32(2):362–375. https://doi.org/10.1002/jgc4.1643

Schaibley VM et al. Limited genomics training among physicians remains a barrier to genomics-based implementation of precision medicine. *Front Med*. 2022;9:757212. https://doi.org/10.3389/fmed.2022.757212

Scheuner MT et al. Delivery of clinical genetic consultative services in the Veterans Health Administration. *Genet Med*. 2014;16(8):609–619. https://doi.org/10.1038/gim.2013.202

Talwar D et al. Genetics/genomics education for nongenetic health professionals: A systematic literature review. *Genet Med*. 2017;19(7):725–732. https://doi.org/10.1038/gim.2016.156

Unim B et al. Current genetic service delivery models for the provision of genetic testing in Europe: A systematic review of the literature. *Front Genet*. 2019;10:552. https://doi.org/10.3389/fgene.2019.00552

White S et al. Mainstreaming genetics and genomics: A systematic review of the barriers and facilitators for nurses and physicians in secondary and tertiary care. *Genet Med*. 2020;22(7):1149–1155. https://doi.org/10.1038/s41436-020-0785-6

Expanded Carrier Screening and Newborn Screening

Josie Pervola, Charlotte Close, and Alexandra Demers

Introduction

For years, carrier screening (CS) has been offered to patients considering future pregnancy or those with an ongoing pregnancy. Historically, gene-by-gene screening was offered for certain conditions in high-risk populations. More recent evidence has shown that panethnic CS is both a more effective and equitable approach, and it is consequently supported by professional societies as an acceptable method of screening along with ethnic-specific and expanded CS. Debate persists, both within and between medical communities, with respect to which conditions to include on CS panels. In addition, there is a discrepancy between contemporary guidelines and conditions included on available panels, with current offerings that are extremely heterogeneous in both size and selection of tested conditions. The discrepancy between contemporary recommendations and the conditions on commercial CS panels presents both pretest and posttest challenges for genetic counselors (GCs).

Similarly, there is significant practice variation in newborn screening (NBS) between and within countries; however, the overarching goal of NBS – early diagnosis and treatment of rare diseases – remains consistent in its aim to impact infant morbidity and mortality. To date, most NBS programs utilize a multiplex testing platform to screen for biomarkers associated with various disorders. Some countries and states then reflex to gene/variant panels and/or next-generation sequencing via a multitiered screening algorithm. Of note, point-of-care events such as hearing screens and congenital heart disease screens can also be included in NBS. Most recently, exome and genome sequencing have become clinically available as diagnostic tools. The integration of these broad analyses into NBS is being considered globally. The ever-evolving practice of NBS illustrates how advancements in science and technology often outpace that of social infrastructure, resulting in many ethical and logistical challenges relevant to GCs. As the number of conditions included in NBS grows and the prospect of genome screening looms on the horizon, pain points with traditional NBS programs will likely be exacerbated and impact genetic counseling practice.

DOI: 10.1201/9781003397847-14

Carrier Screening – Challenges and Strategies

What Size Carrier Screening Panel Is Sufficient to Offer?

A direct correlation exists between the number of conditions included on a CS panel and the detection rate of carriers and at-risk couples (ARCs). Research indicates that the vast majority of ARCs will be captured by screening for conditions with a carrier frequency of $\geq$ 1 in 200, which corresponds to a panel of about 100 conditions. Yet many panels well above this number of conditions are available to patients. Studies have demonstrated a point of saturation, where the percentage of carriers detected plateaus for extremely rare conditions. Modeling indicates that screening for conditions with a carrier frequency of 1/1,000 would yield only two additional couples identified per 10,000 couples screened. At this saturation point, the probability of identifying an ARC in the absence of consanguinity drops below 0.1%, suggesting diminished utility in expanding the panel beyond a certain threshold. Therefore, unless there is an elevated risk due to consanguinity, extensive panels (> 200 conditions) offer limited utility in terms of detection rate.

In addition, using larger panels often means a patient will be a carrier of at least one condition. Identifying carrier individuals, especially during pregnancy, is associated with both emotional and financial consequences. For autosomal recessive (AR) conditions, risk assessment is dependent on the availability of the patient's reproductive partner, and several studies show that partner uptake varies between 42% and 77%. In addition, the number of children conceived with donor sperm or egg has markedly increased over the past 20 years. Often, anonymous sperm or egg donors have more-minimal CS and are not available for updated testing.

GCs may face the "Is more better?" quandary when choosing what type of CS panel to offer in their practice. Patients may come in knowing that testing for hundreds of conditions is available and want "the most comprehensive testing." There are certainly practical aspects of offering testing in clinical practice that we did not discuss here, such as insurance coverage, ease of working with specific laboratories from both a customer service and variant curation perspective, and turnaround time, among others. When having a pretest discussion with patients who are deciding between different sizes of CS panels, utility should be discussed in the context of (1) the presence or absence of consanguinity, (2) if the testing is being performed preconception or prenatally and the psychoemotional impacts of a positive result, and (3) the mode of conception and availability of the partner for testing for precise risk assessment.

Genotype–Phenotype Correlation

Because CS is meant to assess the risk for monogenic disease in a couple's offspring, it is important that screened conditions have a strong gene–disease association; however, this is not the case for some conditions that are included on larger panels. While guidelines provide criteria for conditions suitable for inclusion in CS panels, laboratories can create their own panels, exercising this autonomy as a means of staying competitive. As an example, screening for dihydropyridine dehydrogenase deficiency is currently offered. This is an AR condition that shows large phenotypic variability, ranging from no symptoms to a convulsive disorder with significant motor and intellectual ramifications. There is no correlation between genotype and phenotype. A couple who finds out they are at risk to have a child with this condition based on CS results may face a tremendous amount of uncertainty. A child who is compound heterozygous for the couple's variants may have no symptoms but could also be severely affected. The couple must then decide about pursuing embryo testing, prenatal testing, or postnatal testing, knowing that the relationship between the variants and the phenotype is not certain.

Similarly, when reviewing screening results for a patient or couple, it is vital to investigate the genotype–phenotype relationship when available. Are the couple's variants pathogenic when in trans? Do those specific variants in combination portend a particular phenotype? Many GCs are familiar with conditions like GJB2-related AR nonsyndromic hearing loss, which has well-described genotyping–phenotype correlations. There are also variants with high-allele frequency on panels, such as the p.R229Q NPHS2 variant, that are considered pathogenic only when trans-associated to specific mutations. Variant-specific research is therefore needed prior to disclosing results to patients to confirm that a carrier–carrier couple is at risk to have a symptomatic child and to clarify what the expected phenotype or range of expected phenotypes may be. As patients pursue CS for more and more conditions, foreseeably with population carrier frequencies approaching < 1 in 200, posttest counseling will require more specific research on genotype/phenotype correlation and more counseling about potential uncertainty.

Variant Reporting in Carrier Screening

Laboratories performing CS typically only report on variants classified as pathogenic or likely pathogenic within genes known to be associated with disease. It is important to bear in mind this distinction within the reporting framework, particularly when dealing with a pathogenic variant in trans with a variant of uncertain significance (VUS). For example, if a patient is a carrier for an AR condition and their partner is negative, there may be circumstances in a pregnancy in which the clinical picture warrants an inquiry about the presence or absence of VUSs in the partner who was "negative." Similarly, a child may have a positive newborn screen for an AR condition that was included on CS. It is important to remember that CS is just that – screening. In these circumstances, either prenatally or postnatally, the GC should recontact the performing laboratory to inquire about unreported VUSs in the other member of the couple. Reclassification may be possible in the event of an affected child. These scenarios emphasize the importance of discussing residual risk in posttest counseling.

Similarly, some groups of genetic conditions, such as ciliopathies, are caused by missense variants in larger proportion than other conditions. Missense variants are inherently more difficult to classify using current variant interpretation criteria, and thus, there are more unreported VUSs for this group of conditions when compared to other disorders. As a result, a negative CS result should not preclude inclusion of that condition in a clinician's differential diagnosis when consulting a patient.

Our knowledge of variant pathogenicity is growing in parallel with the diversity and size of genomic databases. We are limited by our current knowledge of disease-causing variants. Additionally, individuals from underrepresented ethnic minorities receive more VUSs due to inadequate representation in genomic databases. When reviewing CS results for a patient or couple, it is important to consider the date the testing was performed. Advances in technology, evolving guidelines, and expanding variant knowledge may necessitate reanalysis or updated testing. In addition, it is imperative that posttest counseling includes a discussion about results being risk reducing and not risk eliminating. GCs and healthcare providers reviewing CS results must assess whether the clinical situation warrants additional follow-up with the performing laboratory to ensure accurate risk assessment and reduce missed diagnoses.

Newborn Screening – Challenges and Strategies

Penetrance and Expressivity

As NBS practices continue to evolve and DNA analysis is more frequently integrated into screening algorithms, challenges with variation in penetrance and expressivity have become apparent. For example, spinal muscular atrophy, Pompe disease, and X-linked adrenoleukodystrophy were added to the American Recommended Universal Screening Panel when novel treatments became commercially available; however, each of these conditions has late-onset variants, in addition to neonatal onset, that don't require treatment in infancy. Consequently, caregivers of asymptomatic infants may face predictive diagnoses which generate a myriad of questions and emotions.

Another example of a condition that can be "diagnosed" asymptomatically via NBS is cystic fibrosis (CF). This occurs through the identification of individuals with one or more VUSs and/or variants of varying clinical consequence (VCC). "VCC" is a term recognized within the CF community to describe variants that have been seen in combination with CF-causing variants in both people with CF and healthy individuals. Individuals who screen positive with at least one of these variants often receive an inconclusive diagnostic determination (CF Screen Positive, Inconclusive Diagnosis), which requires ongoing monitoring due to the possible conversion to a diagnosis of CF based on clinical criteria. The challenge to determine the disease liability of variants requires consideration of functional analysis, population genetics, and clinical information in databases such as CFTR2.

In the context of an uncertain result, either from ambiguous impacts on phenotype or variable expression, genetic counseling for a family of an asymptomatic infant requires nuance and thorough understanding of the condition at hand. Clinical follow-up may require further assessments, such as sweat testing in the case of CF, variant phasing, and/or long-term monitoring. This necessitates a strong partnership between caregivers and clinicians that often relies on mutual acceptance of uncertainty and the utilization of individualized care plans. As long-term data from NBS accumulates, understanding of the true incidence and clinical variability of genetic conditions will begin to emerge. Therefore, GCs must keep abreast of changes in their region's NBS practices and be familiar with literature and variant annotation databases.

The Psychosocial Impacts of a Public Health System

NBS as a public health program intertwines the roles of federal agencies and healthcare providers. This results in GCs being one cog in the large wheel of social infrastructure that caregivers of an infant with an abnormal NBS will encounter. These caregivers have historically expressed frustration that the individuals who notified them of abnormal NBS results lacked adequate knowledge about the condition in question. This is expected, as there are no clear recommendations for who should disclose results of abnormal NBS. The responsibility of disclosure can fall on pediatricians, midwives, receptionists, and so on. Many of these professionals have limited knowledge of genetics and very rarely encounter people affected by any of the conditions on NBS. As a result, recipients of abnormal NBS results are often left devoid of crucial emotional or educational support in a time of significant psychosocial difficulty. Furthermore, in countries like the United States, where NBS is federally mandated and the option to decline screening is not universally offered, pretest education about NBS is only required in about half of states. Consequently, caregivers who receive abnormal NBS results may be shocked with the consequences of a test that they never knew was ordered.

Given that caregivers are likely to interact with people with differing levels of genetic expertise before and after seeing a GC, it's critical that GCs be cognizant of the larger system they're a part of and be mindful of where in the NBS timeline they are meeting caregivers. This will require careful assessment and tailoring of counseling so that each caregiver's informational and psychological needs are met. Follow-up genetic counseling should also be considered because caregivers' priorities are likely to change as they continuously adjust to an abnormal result.

Case Study

A pregnant patient receives a diagnosis of fetal cardiomyopathy at 34 weeks' gestation. The patient and her partner previously pursued CS for 170 conditions earlier in the pregnancy. The patient was found to be a carrier for Pompe disease, and her partner tested negative. The couple was reassured by their provider that they were not an ARC.

The patient delivers at 36 weeks. At birth, the baby screens positive for Pompe disease on NBS. The couple meets with a pediatric GC in the following weeks to follow-up on the positive newborn screening results. The GC notes that the patient was found to be a carrier for Pompe disease via CS and calls the laboratory that performed the couple's testing to inquire about any VUSs for the partner. The GC was informed that the father carries a VUS in the *GAA* gene. The paternal variant was subsequently reclassified to likely pathogenic given their child's enzymatic diagnosis for Pompe disease. The couple went on to pursue an additional pregnancy and chose to conceive via in vitro fertilization with preimplantation genetic testing for monogenic disorders for both *GAA* variants given the 25% recurrence risk.

KEY POINT SUMMARY

- Pretest discussions about CS should include a conversation about the benefits, risks, and limitations of different-sized panels in the context of:
  1. The presence or absence of consanguinity
  2. The timing of the discussion (preconception or prenatal)
  3. The psychoemotional impacts of a positive result
  4. The mode of conception
- Evolution of prenatal or postnatal phenotype may warrant recontacting a CS laboratory about unreported VUSs. This is particularly relevant for AR conditions in which a patient is a known carrier and their partner screened "negative."
- Variant-specific research is necessary prior to discussion of CS and NBS results so that the true risk of symptoms and the expected phenotypic range are fully understood.
- Results of both CS and NBS should be contextualized based on when and where (state, laboratory) testing was performed and what testing methodology was used.

Bibliography

American College of Obstetricians and Gynecologists. Committee opinion 690: Carrier screening in the age of genomic medicine. *Obstet Gynecol.* 2017a;129(3):e35–e40.

American College of Obstetricians and Gynecologists. Committee opinion 691: Carrier screening for genetic conditions. *Obstet Gynecol.* 2017b;129(3):e41–e55.

Arocho R et al. Estimates of donated sperm use in the United States: National survey of family growth 1995–2017. *Fertil Steril.* 2019;112(4):718–723.

Bani M et al. Parents' experience of the communication process of positivity at newborn screening for metabolic diseases: A qualitative study. *Child Care Health Dev.* 2023;49(6):961–971.

Boussaroque A et al. Penetrance is a critical parameter for assessing the disease liability of CFTR variants. *J Cyst Fibros.* 2020;19(6):949–954.

Conway M et al. Pain points in parents' interactions with newborn screening systems: A qualitative study. *BMC Pediatr.* 2022;22(1):167.

Cook S et al. Molecular testing in newborn screening: VUS burden among true positives and secondary reproductive limitations via expanded carrier screening panels. *Genet Med.* 2023:101055.

D'Argenio V. The high-throughput analyses era: Are we ready for the data struggle? *High-Throughput.* 2018;7(1).

DeCelie-Germana JK et al. Diagnostic and communication challenges in cystic fibrosis newborn screening. *Life (Basel).* 2023;13(8).

Enns GM et al. Head imaging abnormalities in dihydropyrimidine dehydrogenase deficiency. *J Inherit Metab Dis.* 2004;27(4):513–522.

Fabiani M et al. Technical factors to consider when developing an expanded carrier screening platform. *Curr Opin Obstet Gynecol.* 2021;33(3):178–183.

Giles Choates M et al. It takes two: Uptake of carrier screening among male reproductive partners. *Prenat Diagn.* 2020;40(3):311–316.

Goldberg JD et al. Expanded carrier screening: What conditions should we screen for? *Prenat Diagn.* 2023;43(4):496–505.

Gregg AR et al. Screening for autosomal recessive and X-linked conditions during pregnancy and preconception: A practice resource of the American College of Medical Genetics and Genomics (ACMG). *Genet Med.* 2021;23(10):1793–1806.

Health Resources & Services Administration. *Recommended Uniform Screening Panel [Internet],* 2023. www.hrsa.gov/advisory-committees/heritable-disorders/rusp

Kawwass JF et al. Trends and outcomes for donor oocyte cycles in the United States, 2000–2010. *JAMA.* 2013;310(22):2426–2434.

Langfelder-Schwind E et al. Practice variation of genetic counselor engagement in the cystic fibrosis newborn screen-positive diagnostic resolution process. *J Genet Couns.* 2019;28(6):1178–1188.

Langfelder-Schwind E et al. Genetic counseling access for parents of newborns who screen positive for cystic fibrosis: Consensus guidelines. *Pediatr Pulmonol.* 2022;57(4):894–902.

McCandless SE, Wright EJ. Mandatory newborn screening in the United States: History, current status, and existential challenges. *Birth Defects Res.* 2020;112(4):350–366.

Mikó Á et al. The mutation-dependent pathogenicity of NPHS2 p.R229Q: A guide for clinical assessment. *Hum Mutat.* 2018;39(12):1854–1860.

National Society of Genetic Counselors. *2023 Professional Status Survey [Internet],* 2023. www.nsgc.org/Research-and-Publications/Professional-Status-Survey

Richards S et al. Standards and guidelines for the interpretation of sequence variants: A joint consensus recommendation of the American College of Medical Genetics and Genomics and the Association for Molecular Pathology. *Genet Med.* 2015;17(5):405–424.

Sagaser KG et al. Expanded carrier screening for reproductive risk assessment: An evidence-based practice guideline from the National Society of Genetic Counselors. *J Genet Couns.* 2023;32(3):540–557.

Simone L et al. Reproductive male partner testing when the female is identified to be a genetic disease carrier. *Prenat Diagn.* 2021;41(1):21–27.

Tluczek A et al. Psychosocial issues related to newborn screening: A systematic review and synthesis. *Int J Neonatal Screen.* 2022;8(4).

Vintschger E et al. Challenges for the implementation of next generation sequencing-based expanded carrier screening: Lessons learned from the ciliopathies. *Eur J Hum Genet.* 2023;31(8):953–961.

Watson MS et al. Newborn screening: Toward a uniform screening panel and system. *Genet Med.* 2006;8(Suppl 1):1S–252S.

Watson MS et al. The progress and future of US newborn screening. *Int J Neonatal Screen.* 2022;8(3).

Westemeyer M et al. Clinical experience with carrier screening in a general population: Support for a comprehensive pan-ethnic approach. *Genet Med.* 2020;22(8):1320–1328.

NAVIGATING NEW FRONTIERS

What Genetic Counselors Need to Know about Genetic Therapies and Clinical Trials

LOUISE BIER AND HETANSHI NAIK

Introduction

The increasing development and availability of therapeutics for rare disorders began in the early 1980s with the Orphan Drug Act (passed into law in 1983) in the United States. This act incentivized drug companies to develop therapeutics for rare disorders by providing tax breaks and market exclusivity for a period after FDA approval. Since then, the development of rare disorder drugs has steadily increased. The field has come a long way since the tragic death of Jesse Gelsinger in 1999, with many genetic therapies in development and several currently FDA approved. These drugs have a range of modalities from small molecules, protein replacement, and antibody therapies to oligonucleotides and cell and gene therapies. The definition of "genetic therapies" has broadened beyond the initial use of viral vectors to transfer genes and now encompasses these as well as gene editing technologies.

Genetic counselors may encounter such therapeutics in a variety of ways and specialties: as clinical genetic counselors informing patients of therapies, as research genetic counselors conducting clinical trials, and as industry genetic counselors working as medical science liaisons or in other roles. Each role interacts with a different aspect of rare disease therapeutics, and the role of genetic counselors in this space will likely continue to expand and diversify. Their skills are uniquely poised to be beneficial to patients, patient advocates, clinicians, industry representatives, and regulatory representatives. Therefore, understanding the challenges genetic counselors may encounter around therapeutics and clinical trials is critical.

Challenges for Clinical Genetic Counselors

Being Broadly Knowledgeable about Therapeutic Technologies to Discuss with Patients

Genetic counselors should have a working understanding of more traditional modalities such as enzyme replacement therapies and substrate reduction therapies while also recognizing newer ones like gene editing, antisense oligonucleotides, and small

DOI: 10.1201/9781003397847-15

interfering RNAs. While a deep understanding of all of these therapies isn't practical, genetic counselors should be aware of the categories of therapies to evaluate and communicate with patients. Review papers on therapies generally include summary tables, which can be key informational resources for genetic counselors. Genetic counselors should also seek out continuing education on these topics.

Navigating Available Information to Identify Appropriate Resources for Clinical Trials or Approved Therapies

Clinical genetic counselors need to be able to critically assess the literature on FDA-approved new therapeutics to discern the potential benefits to their patients and identify ongoing trials their patients may be eligible for. For the latter, the website https://clinicaltrials.gov/ is a key resource for information on available trials. Genetic counselors may then need to help their patients decide if participating in a trial is right for them by discussing its key elements including intensity of the trial, available safety data, potential risks and benefits, and the treatment modality.

Accessing Investigational Drugs outside of a Clinical Trial

In instances where a patient may significantly benefit from a drug that is in clinical trials but cannot participate in the trial (e.g., trial is closed to enrollment), Single Patient Investigational New Drug applications (sINDs), also known as Expanded Access or Compassionate Use, can be sought. These applications request that the FDA grants approval to use an investigational drug for a single patient and can be granted on an expedited basis if there is an urgent need. sINDs are submitted by the treating physician, and clinical genetic counselors can facilitate the process by contacting the pharmaceutical company to determine drug availability through a sIND and then contacting the local Institutional Review Board (IRB) to determine institutional requirements; some IRBs may have modified requirements in emergency cases. This is then followed by the treating physician submitting the sIND request to the FDA (see FDA website for detailed instructions). Clinical genetic counselors may also be involved in the ongoing reporting requirements (e.g., adverse event reporting) once a sIND is established.

Challenges for Research Genetic Counselors

Consenting Patients for Clinical Trials When Risks and Benefits Are Largely Unknown

Consenting patients for interventional clinical trials differs from consent for clinical testing or noninterventional clinical research. While investigational drugs will have cellular and animal models supporting their test use in humans, there may be very little information on the safety profile in humans. The uncertainty of the risk profile may be further complicated by the use of new drug mechanisms where not only the specific investigational drug but the delivery mechanism of the drug are novel or not widely tested across different populations.

The potential benefits of the drug in orphan disease trials will also be largely unknown, may or may not address all aspects of multisystemic diseases, and may impact only certain manifestations of the disease or may not completely resolve particular symptoms. However, even partial improvement of certain symptoms may greatly improve quality of life. Given that rare diseases may have limited long-term natural history data, surrogate endpoints are often used to demonstrate benefits rather than direct measurements of symptoms. For example, a rare disease that is known to be associated with the elevation of a particular biomarker may propose to evaluate efficacy of the drug by a decrease in the biomarker, assuming that this will also be accompanied by a decrease in disease symptomology. However, there may be limited information on precisely how biomarker level correlates with symptom presentation.

When discussing risks/benefits with a patient/caregiver, it is also important to discuss the potential longer-term implications of choosing to participate. Clinical trials may involve a significant time commitment from the patient (and occasionally other family members), frequent study visits, uncomfortable assessments, and restrictions on other aspects of their life (e.g., contraindication of other drugs/foods, birth control requirements, stopping other treatments, etc.).

Navigating the Potential for Therapeutic Misconception

Therapeutic misconception occurs when the line between clinical research and clinical care is blurred and hope of clinical benefit through research becomes an assumption of clinical benefit. Genetic counselors working in rare disease trials must be sensitive to the potential for patients to experience such therapeutic misconception, especially in situations in which there may be no alternative clinical treatments available. The study team must be cognizant that their own hope for a positive clinical trial outcome could potentially feed into therapeutic misconception. Navigating this fine line between hope and therapeutic misconception should be kept in mind throughout the study.

Being Prepared for Psychosocial Aspects That Arise through Clinical Trials

Working with patients in clinical trials requires significant psychosocial preparation, as there are unique psychosocial elements that arise during clinical trials. As described earlier, rare disease clinical trial participation is often intense and requires frequent visits between the study team and patients over years. Genetic counselors may be responsible for monitoring participants' ongoing health and medications, whether related to the rare disease or not. Through these frequent interactions, they often have more insight into participants' lives outside of the trial, both as they support the participant to integrate the clinical trial requirements into their daily lives and simply through the increased interactions with patients. The authors have cared for clinical trial patients as they have gone through weddings and divorces, births and deaths.

Such relationships can be very rewarding, but they also require more vigilance for increased potential for countertransference and emotional overinvestment in the participant's experiences and outcomes during the clinical trial. In some cases, genetic counselors may experience heightened emotions of hope and disappointment based on the participant's course, and prolonged emotional overinvestment may trigger feelings of burnout or psychosocial disengagement. Peer mentoring among other research genetic counselors can assist with balancing psychosocial support and a professional relationship.

Management through Unexpected Trial End

In rare diseases, it is not uncommon for the sponsor to be a relatively small pharmaceutical company with a limited drug pipeline supporting its efforts; should one of its drugs not deliver promising enough results in the timeline expected, studies or entire companies may be shut down with minimal notice, leaving patients who had been participating in the trial without access to a drug that may have been having a positive clinical impact. For genetic counselors involved in such studies, the unexpected closing of a study will require them to navigate the feelings of disappointment, confusion, and lost hope among patients, families, and the study team. Genetic counselors should also be prepared to seek out and advocate for other potential avenues for access to the drug, such as through emergency INDs or Expanded Access Protocols, as discussed earlier.

Challenges for Industry and Patient Advocacy Genetic Counselors

Though not this chapter's focus, it is important to note challenges exist for industry genetic counselors who work in drug development and those who work at patient advocacy groups (PAGs). Industry genetic counselor roles include medical affairs (i.e., medical science liaisons, strategy, patient navigators, etc.) and patient advocacy within biotech/pharmaceutical companies. Common challenges may be outreach to clinical sites for disease educations and to encourage patient identification for trials as well as navigating working with several different PAGs.

Case Study

You are a genetic counselor in a split clinical and research role evaluating and managing patients with lysosomal storage disorders (LSD) and coordinating complex clinical trials for these patients. You see a new patient who is a 5-year-old child with Batten disease (Neuronal Ceroid Lipofuscinosis). The child's current treatment is every 2-week intraventricular infusions of an FDA-approved enzyme replacement therapy (ERT) which is known to slow the loss of ambulation in symptomatic patients. However, it does not treat many of the other symptoms and complications of Batten disease. The parents indicate to you that they are having trouble with the burden of ongoing and lengthy infusions, and they are not seeing the improvement they hoped for in their child.

A new phase I clinical trial of a first-in-human gene therapy using an AAV8 vector for Batten disease was recently initiated at your institution, and you are the primary coordinator for this trial; the patient's treating physician is the PI of the study. You and the physician have a follow-up visit with the child and discuss the trial with the parents. This discussion focuses on:

- *The risks and potential benefits of joining the trial*
  - The ERT infusions would need to be stopped.
  - The gene therapy might not work and might prevent the child from receiving future versions of the gene therapy if modifications are made to the mechanism.
  - There could be an anaphylactic reaction.
  - The child may be the first human to get this experimental drug, so the safety is not known.
- *The complicated logistics of the trial*
  - The screening procedures are complicated and will involve several overnight stays at the hospital, which is at least a 4-hour drive for the parents.
  - The child must stay in the hospital inpatient for 3 days for the study drug administration.
  - Following the administration, there are weekly study visits for the first 2 months, which require specialized lab testing and must be done at the site.
  - The subsequent study visits are a combination of site visits and home visits with a home nursing company.

After this initial discussion, you give the parents a copy of the 35-page consent form and tell them to read it over and think about it. A week later, you have a follow-up telehealth visit with the parents to review the consent form and answer any questions they might have. Their questions are primarily about how quickly improvements will be seen in their child's symptoms if the gene therapy works. You are unable to answer these questions and must emphasize how much is unknown because this is a first-in-human study.

The following week, the parents decide to enroll their child in the trial and seem optimistic about the potential benefits. You schedule all the screening procedures, which include three onsite visits for various imaging procedures and biomarker tests over the course of a month and one home visit for other lab tests. It takes 2 weeks after the screening procedures are completed to get all the results back. Unfortunately, the results show that the child had been previously exposed to an AAV8 and is ineligible for the trial.

You are responsible for calling the parents and breaking this news to them. During the phone call, they express disbelief and anger at finding out their child is not eligible for the trial. They state they were under the assumption their child was already enrolled. You briefly review the consent information about screening procedures with them and explain the purpose of why testing for the AAV8 antibodies prior to dosing of the gene therapy is important for the safety of their child. They express understanding and recall your conversations about the screening visits but are incredibly disappointed. Their child must continue with ERT infusions for the foreseeable future.

As both their research and clinical genetic counselor, you were responsible for the following:

- Giving them information about the current treatment's benefits and limitations
- Giving them information about the gene therapy's benefits and risks
- The complex logistics of the trial
- Helping them decide about enrolling their child in the trial or not
- Supporting them when they learned their child was not eligible for the trial

This example touches on many key aspects and scenarios a genetic counselor involved in gene therapies and clinical trials may experience.

KEY POINT SUMMARY

- genetic counselors should be aware of current and emerging treatment modalities via continuing education.
- Clinical genetic counselors should know how to find clinical trials and how to navigate access both within and outside of clinical trials.
- Research genetic counselors should be aware of the complexities involved with consenting when many risks and benefits are unknown, including the potential for therapeutic misconception.
- Research genetic counselors should be prepared to navigate the unique psychosocial issues that come with serving patients participating in clinical trials.

Bibliography

Approved Cellular and Gene Therapy Products. *The Food and Drug Administration [Internet]*, 2004. www.fda.gov/vaccines-blood-biologics/cellular-gene-therapy-products/approved-cellular-and-gene-therapy-products

Augustine EF et al. Clinical trials in rare disease: Challenges and opportunities. *J Child Neurol.* September 2013;28(9):1142–1150.

ClinicalTrials [Internet]. https://clinicaltrials.gov/

Food and Drug Administration. *For Physicians: How to Request Single Patient Expanded Access ("Compassionate Use") [Internet]*, 2024. www.fda.gov/drugs/investigational-new-drug-ind-application/physicians-how-request-single-patient-expanded-access-compassionate-use

Halley MC et al. Undiagnosed diseases network. Genomics research with undiagnosed children: Ethical challenges at the boundaries of research and clinical care. *J Pediatr.* 2023;261:113537.

Kempf L et al. Challenges of developing and conducting clinical trials in rare disorders. *Am J Med Genet A.* April 2018;176(4):773–783.

Peay HL et al. Expectations and experiences of investigators and parents involved in a clinical trial for Duchenne/Becker muscular dystrophy. *Clin Trials.* February 2014;11(1):77–85.

Reeder R et al. Characterizing clinical genetic counselors' countertransference experiences: An exploratory study. *J Genet Couns.* October 2017;26(5):934–947.

Sibbald B. Death but one unintended consequence of gene-therapy trial. *CMAJ.* 2001; 164(11):1612.

Tambuyzer E et al. Therapies for rare diseases: Therapeutic modalities, progress and challenges ahead. *Nat Rev Drug Discov.* 2020;19(2):93–111.

Tingley K et al. Canadian Inherited Metabolic Diseases Research Network. Stakeholder perspectives on clinical research related to therapies for rare diseases: Therapeutic misconception and the value of research. *Orphanet J Rare Dis.* 2021;16(1):26.

Artificial Intelligence and the Future of Genomic Medicine

Shivani B. Nazareth

Introduction

Artificial intelligence (AI) describes the science and technology of creating machines to "think" like humans. In essence, AI enables computers to simulate tasks that typically require human cognitive function. The concept of AI is not new, but its sophistication has evolved over time. Glimpses of our fascination with this subject date back as early as 700 BC through the Greek mythological story of Talos. A self-moving bronze statue commissioned by Zeus to protect the island of Crete, Talos circled the island three times a day to launch boulders at enemy ships. Talos was a true feat of technological prowess, revered for its human-like skills. Since then, incredible strides in AI have led to self-driving cars, conversational chatbots, and clinical decision support tools that evoke a similar sense of awe. By bridging gaps in patient care and augmenting patient–provider interactions, AI is poised to change medicine as we know it.

Making Sense of AI

Before delving into clinical use cases of AI, it's important to understand the terminology used to describe this science. A fundamental subtype of AI is **machine learning**, whereby computers perform tasks without being explicitly programmed to do so. Machine learning systems are trained on large sets of data, which, in turn, allow computers to identify patterns and make predictions. A simple example of machine learning is text autocompletion. Type the word "good," and the next-most-likely words surface, including "morning" or "job." Pattern recognition is at the heart of machine learning systems. **Deep learning** is a form of machine learning through which computers use artificial neural networks to predict more complex patterns. Deep learning networks draw inspiration from the neural networks of the human brain. See Figure 16.1.

A pivotal breakthrough in AI technology is the ability of machines to interpret and respond to human language – rather than computer language – in a meaningful way, referred to as **natural language processing** (NLP). NLP requires translating and mapping words into concepts. Virtual assistants, such as Apple's Siri, use NLP

DOI: 10.1201/9781003397847-16

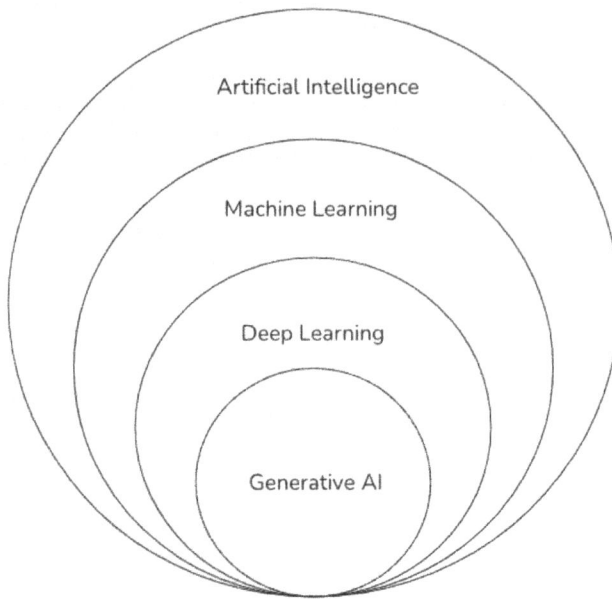

Figure 16.1   The subtypes of AI.

to translate spoken words into commands, search the internet or your phone, and respond to a given prompt. Most recently, NLP capabilities have expanded to include writing complex text, summarizing articles, and creating social media posts on a variety of specialty topics, including finance, healthcare, and law. Behind the scenes, NLP capabilities rely on **large language models** (LLMs) to generate refined patterns of text, also called **generative AI**. Recent examples of LLMs that have gained significant attention include ChatGPT, Gemini, PaLM, and LLaMA.

Algorithms That Learn

The data-intensive nature of medicine makes it a prime candidate for the use of AI and deep learning algorithms. Studies have already demonstrated the performance of generative AI to be on par with physicians in responding to common patient questions or classifying medical images. For example, a comparison of ophthalmologists and LLM chatbot responses to 200 questions found that the LLM was able to appropriately respond to written questions. There were some incorrect medical responses; however, the overall potential harm of AI-generated medical advice did not differ significantly from human medical advice. Data collected from online health forums have also found that LLM chatbots can generate more empathetic responses to questions.

In 2023, ChatGPT made headlines for its ability to pass the United States Medical Licensing Exam (USMLE), excluding questions with images or sounds. This is astounding in that large language models appear to be able to self-learn without explicit training. Known as "in-context" learning, these algorithms rely on smaller machine-learning models to train. These capabilities are relevant to advancing genomics and precision medicine for rare diseases. Using NLP and deep learning, clinicians and researchers can query large volumes of patient data that already exist within electronic health records (EHRs) to make population risk predictions, intervene at earlier stages of disease, and improve healthcare outcomes.

Applications and Challenges of AI in Genomics

Identifying Undiagnosed Patients   Medical data should ideally be structured and searchable as discrete values within EHRs using variable names, such as age, weight, blood pressure, or medication doses, each of which corresponds to a specific value. In reality, medical documentation is complex and often unstructured, existing in multimodal formats like handwritten physician notes, PDF lab reports with genomic findings, and even images, like a pedigree or x-ray. It is therefore time-consuming to review a patient's medical history in its entirety. Further complicating matters, different medical specialties require unique data points and expertise.

AI-enhanced EHRs have the potential to help clinicians scan medical records holistically and display diagnostic possibilities much faster than any individual person. As an example, AI could flag patients with a personal and family history consistent with a genetic syndrome and then suggest a list of clinically relevant tests for confirmation. Such tools could help primary care and other nongenetic providers identify patients who would benefit from genetic counseling and/or testing. Going one step further, AI trained on large datasets of genomic information can shorten time to diagnosis, accurately narrow down variants related to a specific phenotype, and potentially accelerate drug development models for otherwise "orphan" diseases. Similarly, AI shows promise in the ability to recognize patterns within large patient cohorts and use it to find appropriate clinical trials. That said, the quality of data within the EHR greatly influences the accuracy of the output, highlighting the fact that patient care is nuanced and that medicine is not simply a transactional exchange but also an art. A healthy balance of trust and human judgment will be necessary to ensure that AI-generated clinical decision support is not deployed as a blind substitute for subject matter expertise.

Scaling Genetic Services   Genetic counseling plays a crucial role in empowering individuals and families to make informed decisions regarding their genetic health. As the field advances, integration of AI has emerged as a promising tool to augment the practice of genetic counseling. In clinical settings, one study found that only 20% of a genetic counselor's time is spent with the patient. A large percentage of time is devoted to patient-related activities such as letter writing, administrative tasks, and case preparation, all of which are prime use cases for AI technology.

An AI-supported chatbot named Gia, or Genetic Information Assistant, has been utilized in mammography and obstetric settings to triage patients who would benefit from hereditary cancer genetic testing. Developed by software engineers and genetic counselors, Gia ingests patients' family history information via a web-based application and maps it against established medical guidelines for cancer risk assessment, including the National Comprehensive Cancer Network (NCCN) and Tyrer-Cuzick criteria. When Gia was deployed in advance of routine women's health exams, nearly 90% of patients completed the questionnaire, and 25% met the NCCN criteria for genetic testing. Gia demonstrated the ability to accurately identify and educate patients who met criteria for genetic testing. This allowed nongenetics experts and clinicians with limited access to a genetic counselor to offer testing to patients at risk for hereditary breast and ovarian cancer syndrome. Using an AI-supported chatbot to triage patients into risk categories would allow genetic counselors to focus on cases in which nuanced expertise is required, allowing them to practice at the top of their license.

Ambient Transcription   While direct patient care is a source of great satisfaction for many clinicians, there is well-documented burnout associated with having to log all patient encounters within EHRs. Ambient artificial intelligence – technology that uses a microphone to transcribe conversations in real time directly into an EHR – is perhaps the most practical use case of AI in healthcare. This technology relies on machine learning, NLP, and clinical training to ensure proper formatting. Figure 16.2 from AWS HealthScribe illustrates the potential for ambient AI to reduce the amount of time a provider would have to spend on documentation. Instead, the provider can simply read the note and edit or supplement it to ensure accuracy.

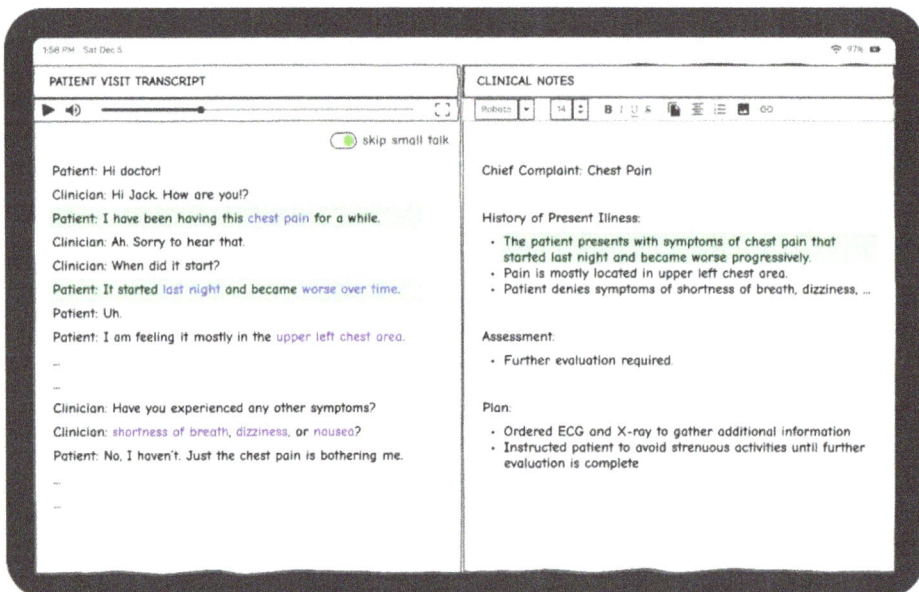

Figure 16.2   Illustrative example of the application experience that healthcare developers can provide users with AWS HealthScribe. (From Mark et al. 2023, with permission.)

Initial responses from providers and patients who have agreed to utilize an AI scribe have been enthusiastic. In one study facilitated at the Permanente Medical Group, 81% of patients reported that their doctors spent less time looking at the computer screen than in previous visits. All patients reported feeling "neutral" to "very comfortable" about ambient transcription and said it had no effect or enhanced their visit. A total of 3,442 clinicians and staff used the AI scribe; physicians noted meaningful and more effective interactions with patients as well as a reduction in after-hours work. It is by no means a complete replacement for human documentation. The study noted a few instances of AI hallucination, for example a physician saying that a patient needed to schedule a prostate exam but the AI scribe summarizing that the exam had already occurred. One can imagine that such transcription for a genetic counseling session may also involve more training on family history documentation and human review of clinical findings to ensure accuracy.

Keeping Up with AI   As AI advances, clinicians must be willing to drive responsible utilization within their respective work environments. For genetic counselors, this could mean piloting new AI tools for patient education or medical documentation. AI may change the way genetic counselors interact with patients, just as earlier technologies like telemedicine disrupted the model of face-to-face sessions. AI will broaden access to genetic information, but human expertise will be necessary to ensure clinical integrity, responsible oversight, and equity within healthcare settings. Genetic counselors who are willing to experiment, adopt, critique, and embrace AI are more likely to thrive as the technology continues to evolve.

Real-World Example

Leveraging AI to augment clinical decisions has potential to remove the diagnostic odyssey that plagues many families with rare diseases. Dr. Dave is a pediatrician at a solo practice in rural Illinois. In a comment to *JAMA* in September 2023, he wrote the following.

> *Yesterday I saw a child with [a] variety of features characteristic of a genetic syndrome. I asked to chatGPT for a diagnosis and it came out within seconds with Rubinstein–Taybi syndrome. Astounding and overwhelming. Further, it suggested all the tests I would need, putting cAMP-response element binding protein (CREBBP) genome assay as the most desired. The child at a very young age has been seen by a geneticist at a tertiary center and the tests done did not include CREBBP genome sequence. The technology is a godsend for rural physicians like me because the nearest tertiary center is about 90 miles away and rural America is like the developing world within America.*

Shifting genomics into general medicine – including pediatrics, primary care, obstetrics, and cardiology – requires clinicians to routinely and promptly identify patients who can benefit from a genetic evaluation. In reality, this does not occur consistently. This real-world example underscores the potential of AI-assisted technologies to accelerate the time to diagnosis for patients with rare diseases and remove existing barriers to genetic testing. A more holistic view of patient care can emerge with such tools, including the development of longitudinal care plans with multiple specialists and cascade testing for at-risk relatives. With this in mind, AI may in fact be the technology that finally supports the integration of genomics into routine medicine, allowing patients and their families to fully realize the benefit of early diagnosis, intervention, and ultimately disease prevention.

KEY POINT SUMMARY

- The data-intensive nature of genomics makes it a prime candidate for the use of AI.
- Deployed across electronic health records, AI may help primary care and other nongenetic experts identify patients who require genetic counseling and/or testing.
- Leveraging AI to augment clinical decisions has potential to remove the diagnostic odyssey that plagues many families with rare diseases.
- A healthy balance of trust and human judgment will be necessary to ensure that AI-generated clinical decision support is not deployed as a blind substitute for subject matter expertise.

Bibliography

Attard CA et al. Genetic counselor workflow study: The times are they a-changin'? *J Genet Couns*. 2019;28(1):130–140.

Ault A. AI bot ChatGPT passes US medical licensing exams without cramming – Unlike students. *Medscape*, 2023. www.medscape.com/viewarticle/987549?form=fpf

Ayers JW et al. Comparing physician and artificial intelligence chatbot responses to patient questions posted to a public social media forum. *JAMA Intern Med*. 2023;183(6):589–596.

Barz B et al. Diverse perspectives on the relationship between artificial intelligence and pattern recognition. Centre for Pattern Recognition and Machine Intelligence. *Front Patt Recogn Artif Intell*. 2019:23–34.

Bernstein IA et al. Comparison of ophthalmologist and large language model chatbot responses to online patient eye care questions. *JAMA Netw Open*. 2023;6(8):e2330320.

Chary M et al. A review of natural language processing in medical education. *West J Emerg Med*. 2019;20(1):78–86.

ChatGPT. https://openai.com/index/chatgpt/

Gaube S et al. Do as AI say: Susceptibility in deployment of clinical decision-aids. *NPJ Digit Med*. 2021;4(1):31.

Harris JE. An AI-enhanced electronic health record could boost primary care productivity. *JAMA*. 2023;330(9):801–802.

Kauf C et al. Event knowledge in large language models: The gap between the impossible and the unlikely. *Cogn Sci.* 2023;47:e13386.

Kulkarni PA, Singh H. Artificial intelligence in clinical diagnosis: Opportunities, challenges, and hype. *JAMA.* 2023;330(4):317–318.

Mark J et al. *Introducing AWS HealthScribe [Internet]*, 2023. https://aws.amazon.com/blogs/industries/industries-introducing-aws-healthscribe/

Nazareth S et al. Hereditary cancer risk using a genetic chatbot before routine care visits. *Obstet Gynecol.* 2021;138(6):860–870.

Quiroz JC et al. Challenges of developing a digital scribe to reduce clinical documentation burden. *NPJ Digit Med.* 2019;2:114.

Shashkevich A. Stanford researcher examines earliest concepts of artificial intelligence, robots in ancient myths. *Stanford Report [Internet]*, 2019. https://news.stanford.edu/2019/02/28/ancient-myths-reveal-early-fantasies-artificial-life/

Snir M et al. Democratizing genomics: Leveraging software to make genetics an integral part of routine care. *Am J Med Genet C.* 2021;187C:14–27.

Tierney G et al. Ambient artificial intelligence scribes to alleviate the burden of clinical documentation. *NEJM Catal Innov Care Deliv.* 2024;5(3).

Vilhekar RS, Rawekar A. Artificial intelligence in genetics. *Cureus.* 2024;16(1):e52035.

Zewe A. Large language models in context learning. *MIT News [Internet]*, 2023. news.mit.edu/2023/large-language-models-in-context-learning-0207

Index

Note: Page numbers in *italics* indicate a figure and page numbers in **bold** indicate a table on the corresponding page.

A

AAV8 vector, for Batten disease, 98, 99
Accreditation Council for Genetic
    Counseling (ACGC), 46
All of Us study, 15
American Academy of Pediatrics (AAP), 64
American College of Medical Genetics (ACMG)
    ACMG/AMP criteria, 1, 5, 52, 64
    carrier screening guidelines, 11
    and EHR, 51
    family studies, 3–4
    secondary findings, 15, 18
American College of Obstetricians and
    Gynecologists (ACOG), 11, 25
APOL1 high-risk genotype, 83, 84
artificial intelligence (AI)
    ambient transcription, 104–105
    and deep learning, 101–103
    defined, 101
    example, 105–106
    genetic counseling, 103, 105
    in genomics, 103–105
    integration with EHR systems, 51
    subtypes of, 101–102, *102*
    tools for patient education or medical
        documentation, 105

Ashkenazi Jewish (AJ) descent, 10, 11
assent, 64–65, *see also* consent, acute settings;
    informed consent
Association for Molecular Pathology (AMP),
    1, 51
associative countertransference, 37, *see also*
    countertransference
at-risk couples (ARCs), 88
autosomal recessive (AR), 60, 66, 88
AWS HealthScribe, 104, *104*

B

Baby Boomers (1946–1964), 45
body mass index (BMI), 11
BRCA1 variant, 41, 54

C

cardiomyopathy gene, 16
carrier screening (CS)
    ACMG guidelines for cystic fibrosis, 11
    challenges and strategies, 88–90
    genotype–phenotype correlation, 88–89
    panel size, 88
    partner, 54, 61
    variant reporting, 89–90

cell-free DNA (cfDNA), 11
CFTR2, 90
ChatGPT, 102
clinical genetic counselors, *see also* research
    genetic counselors
  resources for clinical trials or approved
    therapies, 95
  therapeutic technologies, 94–95
Clinical Genome Resource (ClinGen), 1, 3–5
Clinical Laboratory Improvement
    Amendments (CLIA), 15, 17–19
ClinVar, 3
College of American Pathologists (CAP), 1
continuing medical education (CME), 82
consent, acute settings, *see also* informed
    consent; minors, genetic testing of
  adults without capacity, 71
  case study, 71–72
  challenges and strategies, 68–71
  genetic testing, 69–70
  loss of control/unpredictability, 68–69
  time pressure, 70–71
countertransference
  associative, 37
  case study, 41
  challenges and strategies, 39–41
  common causes of, 39
  consequences, 40–41
  identifying signs of, 39
  impact of, 40–41
  projective, 37
  self-awareness and, 37
  types of, 37–38
COVID pandemic, 47, 78, 81
CYP2C19, 19
cystic fibrosis (CF), 11, 61, 90

D

Deciphering Developmental Disorders
    Study (DDD), 5
deep learning, 101–103, *see also* artificial
    intelligence (AI)
*Diagnostic and Statistical Manual of Mental
    Disorders* (Fifth Edition), 33
diversity, equity, inclusion, and justice
    (DEIJ), 47–48
Dual-Process Model (Stroebe and Schut),
    31, *31*

E

electronic health record (EHR)
  adoption rates, 51
  advantages of, 53
  AI-enhanced, 103, 104
  challenges and strategies, 52–55
  clinical care, 52–54
  documentation in, 51–54
  ethical/legal issues, 55
  family member records, 54
  genomic data use, 51, 52
  patient data, 103
  technical challenges, 52
ethical issues, for predictive genetic testing
  case study, 78
  challenges and strategies, 74–77
  informed consent for, *see* informed
    consent
exome or genome sequencing (ES/GS), 2, 4

F

Fast Healthcare Interoperability Resources
    (FHIR), 52
frontotemporal dementia (FTD), 74

G

GAA gene, 92
GeneMatcher, 5
Generation X (1965–1980), 45
Generation Z (Gen Z; 1997–2012), 44–45,
    47
generative AI, 102
genes of uncertain significance (GUS), 5
Genetic Information Assistant (Gia),
    103–104
Genome Aggregation Database (gnomAD),
    3, 4
genomic testing
  bias in guidelines and practice in genetics,
    10–12
  case study, 12–13
  challenges and strategies, 9–12
  lack of diversity in, 10
  REA in, *see* race, ethnicity, and
    ancestry
  SDOH (social determinants of health), 8

H

HBB carriers, 11
Health Information Technologies for Economic and Clinical Health (HITECH), 51
HTT gene, 74
Human Gene Mutation Database (HGMD), 3
Huntington's disease (HD), 74
hypertrophic cardiomyopathy (HCM), 25, 71, 83

I

informed consent, *see also* consent, acute settings; minors, genetic
    in absence of significant other or support person, 75–76
    family member's genetic status, 75
    for genetic testing, 76–77
    in presence of cognitive or psychiatric symptoms, 74–75
    in presence of family coercion, 77
Institutional Review Board (IRB), 95
interpreters
    ad hoc *vs.* professional, 57–58
    case study, 61
    challenges and strategies, 57–61
    cultural barriers, 59
    education, 59–61
    miscommunication, 58–59

K

Kübler-Ross model, 28

L

large language models (LLMs), 102
limited English proficiency (LEP), 57, 60
long-QT syndrome (LQTS), 83
loss and grief in counseling, 28–32
lysosomal storage disorders (LSD), 98

M

machine learning, 101, 103, 104
Matchmaker Exchange, 5
Millennials (1981–1996), 44–45

minors, genetic testing of
    assessing, 63–64
    case study, 66
    informed consent *vs.* assent, 64–65
    results disclosure and follow-up, 65–66
motivational interviewing (MI), 24
MyGene2, 5
MYH7 gene, 25, 54

N

National Comprehensive Cancer Network (NCCN), 24, 104
National Society of Genetic Counselors (NSGC), 66, 76, 80
natural language processing (NLP), 101–104
neonatal intensive care unit (NICU), 71, 72
newborn screening (NBS)
    challenges and strategies, 90–91
    penetrance and expressivity, 90–91
    psychosocial impacts of public health system, 91
    variation in, 87
next-generation sequencing (NGS), 15
nondirectiveness, 22–23
    best-practice guidelines, 23–25
    case study, 25–26
    challenges and strategies, 21–25
    inadvertent directiveness, 22–23
    inevitable directiveness, 23
    positive relationship-building, 21–22
noninvasive genetic screening (NIPS), 22, 26, 71

P

polygenic risk scores (PRS), 12
preimplantation genetic testing for aneuploidy (PGT-A), 25
projective countertransference, 37, *see also* countertransference
PubMed, 5

R

race, ethnicity, and ancestry (REA)
    data collection, 9, 10, 12
    definition, **9**
    in genomic testing, 8
    guidelines and practice in genetics, 10–12

race/ethnicity-based screening, 9
RAC1 gene, 5
rapid genome sequencing (rGS), 71
reciprocal engagement model (REM), 24, 25
recreational genetics, 44
research genetic counselors, 94–95, 99,
        see also clinical genetic counselors
    consenting patients for clinical trials,
        95–96
    management through unexpected trial
        end, 97
    navigating potential for therapeutic
        misconception, 96
    psychosocial aspects through clinical
        trials, 96–97
research genetic testing
    case study, 19
    CLIA-certified laboratory, 16–17
    counseling, 15–16
    outdated research genetic report
        findings, 17
    study design, 18

S

Sequence Variant Interpretation Working
    Group (SVI WG), 1
Shared decision-making (SDM), 24, 60
Single Patient Investigational New Drug
    applications (sINDs), 95
social determinants of health (SDOH), 8
    specialties, genetic, 80, 81–84
student training
    case study, 48
    challenges and strategies, 45–48
    generational gap in learning and teaching,
        45–46
    with genetic and genomic technologies, 46
    genetic counseling graduate program
        network, 48
    genetic counseling students, 44–45

increasing access to, 46–47
    promoting DEIJ, 47–48

T

Tasks of Mourning (Worden), 31, *31*
telemedicine, 47, 51, 81, 105
Trans-Omics for Precision Medicine
    (TOPMed), 3

U

United States Medical Licensing Exam
    (USMLE), 102
USH2 gene, 66

V

variant of uncertain significance (VUS), 92
    case study, 5–6
    challenges and strategies, 2–5
    ClinGen, 3
    de novo variant, 3
    discrepancies in classifications, 2
    follow-up, 4
    genetic diagnoses, 10
    gene transcript number, 2
    human genome reference build, 2
    inherited or familial variant, 3–4
    pathogenic variants, 89
    public databases, 3
    reclassification, 4–5
    researching a variant, 2–5
    variants in GUS, 5
    tools for transcripts, 2
varying clinical consequence (VCC), 90

W

whole-exome sequencing (WES), 66
workplace-based assessments (WBAs), 46